the Total Detox plan

The Total Detox Plan reports information and opinions
of medical and other professionals which may be of
general interest to the reader. It is advisory only and
is not intended to serve as a medical textbook or other
procedural guidebook for either physicians or patients.
The information and opinions contained herein, which
should not be used or relied upon without consultation
and advice of a physician, are those solely of the author
and not those of the publishers who disclaim any
responsibility for the accuracy of such information and
opinions and any responsibility for any consequences
that may result from any use or reliance thereon by
the reader.

THIS IS A CARLTON BOOK

Text © Dr Sarah Brewer 2000
Design © Carlton Books Limited 2000

This edition published by Carlton Books Limited 2004
20 Mortimer Street
London
W1N 7RD

A CIP catalogue record for this book is available from the
British Library

ISBN 1 85868 928 7

Project Editor: Camilla MacWhannell
Editor: Trish Burgess
Art Direction: Diane Spender
Design: Dave Jones
Picture Research: Prudence Korda
Production: Garry Lewis

Printed and bound in Dubai

Dr Sarah Brewer M.A., M.B., B.Chir **Columnist for the Daily Telegraph**

the Total Detox plan

A comprehensive programme to cleanse your mind and body

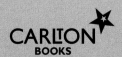

CARLTON
BOOKS

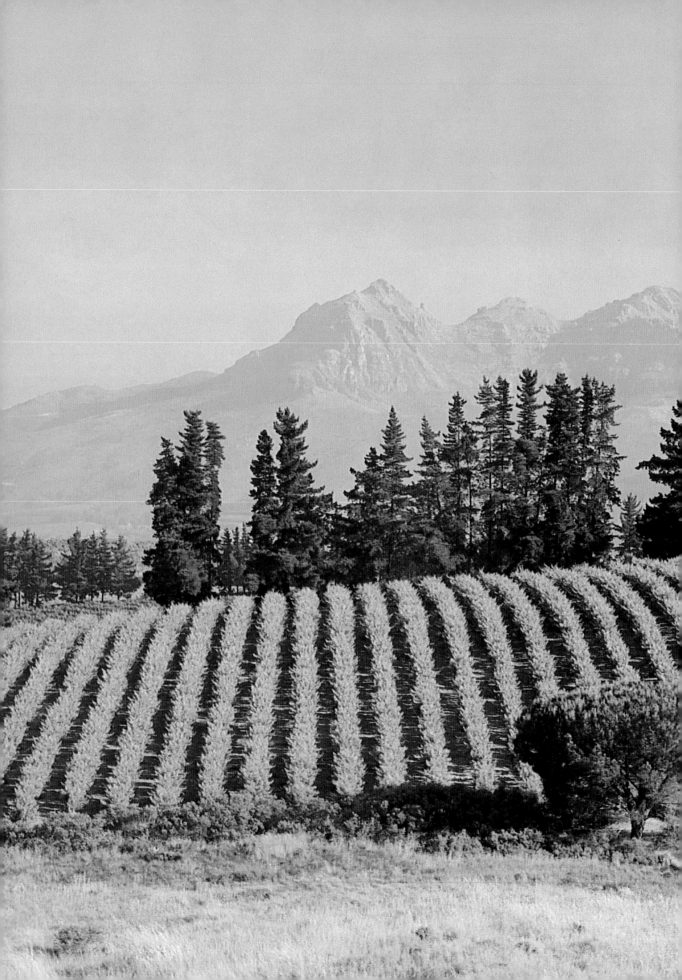

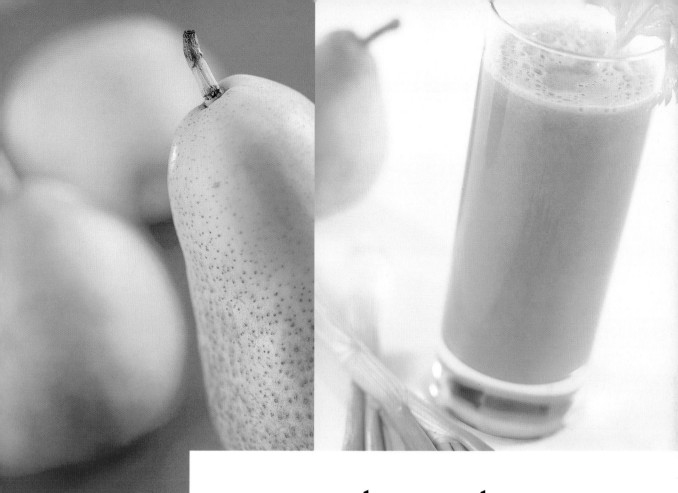

contents

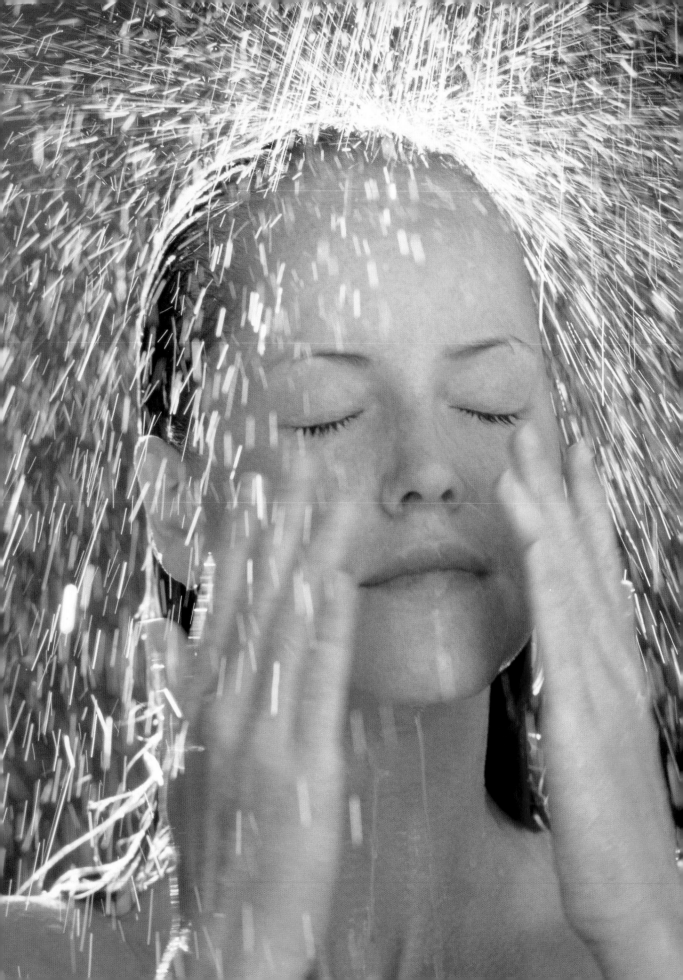

introduction

Detox is a popular technique to help you address an unhealthy diet and lifestyle. Although modern science underlines the principles involved, it is based on ancient practices found in many cultures throughout the world.

The decision to detox may be triggered by a desire to lose weight and get fit, or in response to symptoms of sluggishness, lacking in energy, recurrent infections or difficulty coping with excess stress. Other people just wake up one morning and feel unhealthy, suffering from a coated tongue, bad breath, lacklustre skin and a profound need to start the first day of the rest of their life by ridding their body, diet and environment of as many toxins as possible.

Detox is a simple, two-stage process of cleansing, followed by nutritional balancing. There is no need to follow a rigorous regime of fasting and extreme self-denial. In fact, this may even be harmful by releasing too many toxins, too quickly. It is preferable to follow a simple, pleasurable yet healthy diet containing fresh, wholesome and organic juices, fruit, vegetables, saladstuff, pulses, wholegrain cereals, live bio yoghurt, cottage cheese, fish and chicken. Vegetables can be made into nourishing soups or served lightly steamed and even raw and crunchy where appropriate.

A variety of herbal remedies help to boost the elimination of toxins from your body and, once the cleansing process is underway, a balancing programme is started to improve your overall nutrition, correct dietary deficiencies and to support the detoxification plan.

Complementary techniques such as massage, skin brushing, hydrotherapy, meditation, homeopathy, acupuncture and aromatherapy can also be used throughout the detox process.

This book will help you assess your need for detoxification, and guide you through the important cleansing and balancing stages to achieve the desirable benefits such as improved immunity to infection and a renewed zest for life. And to make the whole process more enjoyable, it shows you how to use a variety of techniques to help you feel more energized, relaxed and indulged as your overall health improves.

Dr Sarah Brewer

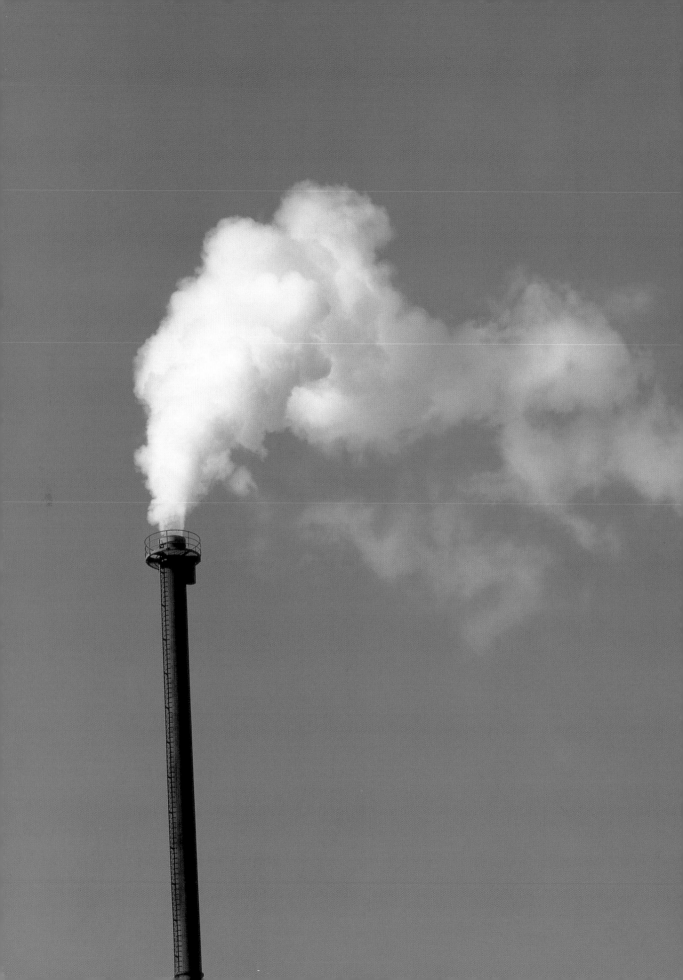

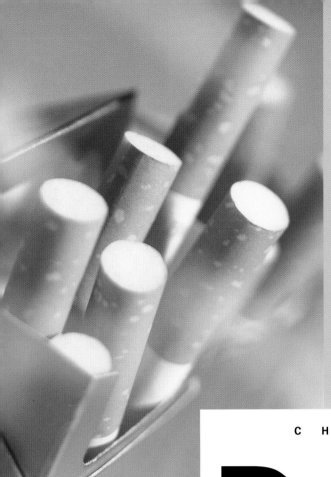

Detoxing – removing harmful substances from the body – is something everyone feels the need to do from time to time. It is the basis of all those New Year resolutions relating to health: becoming fitter, cutting back on alcohol, giving up smoking, going organic...

CHAPTER ONE

why Detox?

However, instead of regarding detox as an occasional health-boosting programme, it should ideally become a way of life. Detox helps to rid the body of potentially harmful chemicals, as well as improving the function of important elimination organs such as the liver, kidneys, intestinal tract and skin. It is especially vital for people under stress, or those who feel tired all the time, run down, have a low immunity to illness, or a tendency towards allergies, headaches, dry, itchy skin, increased mucus production and poor concentration.

We live in a toxic world, and every day we are bombarded by harmful chemicals from our diet, lifestyle, the environment around us and even as a by-product of our own metabolism and the medications we take.

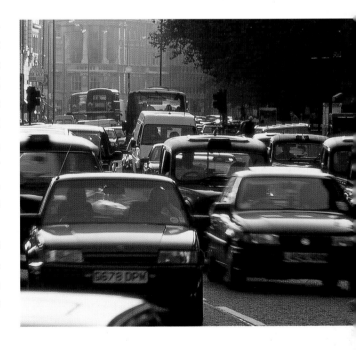

Detoxification

Detoxification is the body's natural process of neutralizing toxins and preparing them for elimination from the body through the actions of the liver, kidneys, bowels, lungs and sweat glands in the skin.

Most people are aware that their diet needs improving, whether by cutting out so-called junk foods, eating more fruit and vegetables, reducing intake of salt, sugar and caffeine, or obtaining a better balance of omega-3 and omega-6 fats and saturated fats. Many of us also know that our lifestyle habits could be improved by taking more exercise, avoiding cigarette smoke and cutting back on drugs of abuse, including alcohol.

It is estimated that every year Western adults are exposed to over 6 kg (13 lb) of food additives, colourings, flavourings, preservatives, waxes and agrochemicals, such as fertilizers, growth enhancers, pesticides and herbicide residues. These all have toxic effects on humans, and the Environment Protection Agency in the United States considers that 60 per cent of all herbicides, 90 per cent of all fungicides and 30 per cent of all insecticides are potentially cancer-causing.

We are also surrounded by atmospheric pollutants, such as chlorofluorocarbons, acid rain, industrial gases and exhaust fumes. Toxic metals, including lead, aluminium and cadmium, are widespread in our environment and some, such as mercury, even reside in the mouth (from the fillings in our teeth).

Every time you inhale cigarette smoke – even if it belongs to someone else – you are exposed to around 4,000 chemicals, of which a significant number are known to be carcinogenic. Unfiltered drinking water from your tap contains traces of almost 1,000 chemicals, while over 10,000 artificial chemicals are added to our food to improve its growth, appearance and storage qualities. Very few of these are intended to enhance nutritional value.

The liver is the most important internal organ for detoxifying the body. While it has amazing powers of regeneration, its enzyme functions are frequently overloaded by a poor, rich or fatty diet, and excess alcohol intake. This produces a variety of symptoms, including bloating, flatulence, lack of energy and fatigue – all symptoms that can improve significantly by following a detox programme.

Organs of detoxification

The skin is the largest detox organ and has important eliminatory functions. Increasing numbers of people suffer from inflammatory skin conditions, such as acne, eczema, psoriasis and skin infections, or the skin might simply appear dingy. Clarity, texture and appearance are readily improved by detoxification, making the skin seem literally to glow with health.

The intestinal tract also has important eliminatory actions, yet disorders such as irritable bowel syndrome, dysbiosis (abnormal bacterial balance) and constipation are widespread.

What does detox do?

Detox brings with it a number of desirable benefits, including improved health and immunity, mental clarity, extra energy and vitality. Skin will become clearer, bowels more regular and liver and kidney function more efficient. As a result, the risk of modern illnesses, such as stress reactions, inflammatory conditions, coronary heart disease, recurrent infections, hormone imbalances, impaired fertility and even cancer, will be reduced.

Detox involves starting a long-term programme to rid your body of toxins through relatively simple dietary changes. If you wish, you can fast for a day or two at the beginning, but this isn't obligatory and is actually inadvisable for some people. It might also contribute to the toxic load by stressing the body and liberating a large number of free radicals, which are harmful by-products of metabolism that can damage cells and genetic material, and toxins stored in fatty (adipose) tissues. It is therefore best to avoid a true water-only fast, and instead to follow a juice-fast, or to eat a simple diet of organic fruit, vegetables and wholegrain cereals, such as steamed brown rice. Taking a variety of vitamin, mineral and herbal supplements is also

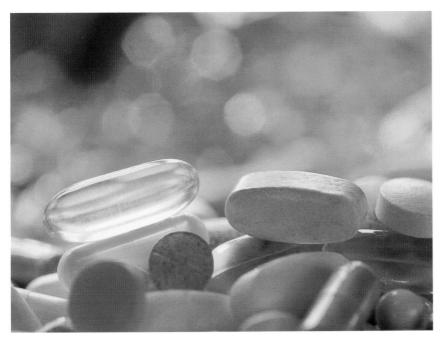

Above: *A variety of supplements can aid the total detox cleansing process*

Having chosen the dietary and lifestyle changes, and the cleansing or nutritive supplements you wish to take, the next step is to decide which complementary therapies to include in your detox programme. The most popular are massage, skin brushing, hydrotherapy, meditation, homoeopathy, acupuncture, aromatherapy and colonic irrigation. A sauna or steam room session to promote sweating and elimination of toxins through the skin is also beneficial for some people.

helpful in boosting the elimination of toxins. While cleansing the body, they can also help to improve general nutrition, correct dietary deficiencies, support the body's natural detoxification processes and improve immunity.

Few of us obtain adequate amounts of protective antioxidants, such as vitamins A, C and E, from our diet, and those we do acquire often work inefficiently at detoxifying free radicals because we lack zinc. A significant number of men are zinc deficient as 5 mg – one third of the adult daily requirement – is lost in each ejaculation. It is, however, relatively easy to test for and correct zinc deficiency (see page 56). More worrying – and more widespread – is lack of selenium, the most important antioxidant mineral. In Britain, for example, average selenium intakes have almost halved over the last 20 years, from 60 mcg to 34 mcg per day. Those with the lowest selenium intakes have the highest risk of developing leukaemia or cancers of the colon, rectum, stomach, breast, ovary, pancreas, prostate gland, bladder, skin and lungs. A randomized study of 1,312 patients showed that those receiving 200 mcg of selenium a day had a 52 per cent lower risk of dying from cancer than those receiving a placebo. As a result, the trial was stopped early so that everyone could benefit from taking selenium supplements.

While everyone will benefit from detox, it is not always plain sailing. Withdrawal from some chemicals, such as caffeine, can cause transient irritability, and elimination of other toxins can cause brief symptoms such as pimples or a coated tongue. This is more likely to occur if you try to detox too quickly – by going on a water-only fast, for example. It is easier and more pleasant to take things slowly, eating a simple diet and drinking mineral water plus a selection of juices.

You should attempt detox only if you feel relatively fit and well. If you are ill, convalescing or taking prescribed medications, do not start a full detox programme unless your doctor is happy to sanction it. Instead, make changes so that your diet and lifestyle are generally more healthy. This could include taking a general nutritional supplement of A–Z vitamins and minerals, an antioxidant preparation containing selenium plus vitamins A, C and E, and evening primrose oil for essential fatty acids.

Avoid full detox when you are pregnant or breast-feeding. Instead, eat a healthy diet, avoid cigarette smoke and alcohol altogether, and take a good multivitamin and mineral supplement especially designed for pregnancy, plus a specially balanced essential fatty acid formula based on evening primrose oil and DHA (docosahexaenoic acid) derived from fish oils and/or algae extracts.

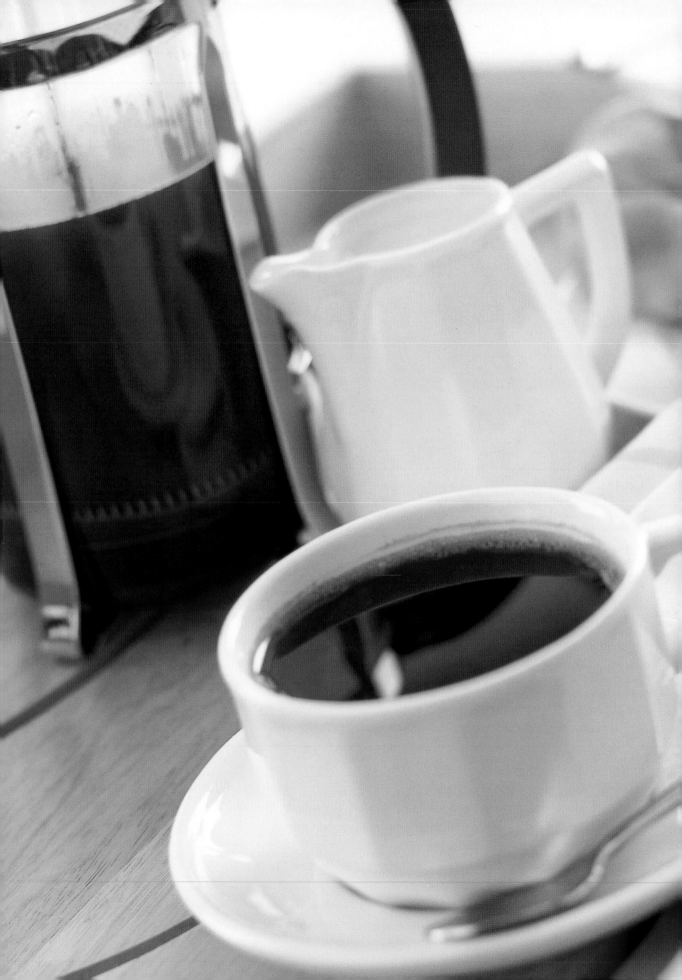

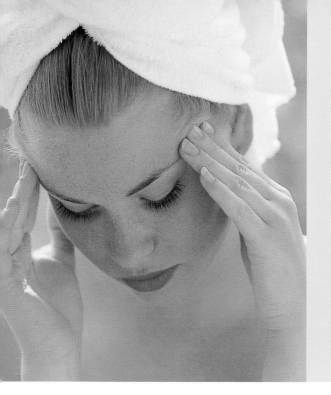

Detoxification is your body's way of ridding itself of unwanted chemicals. These might result from your own metabolism, or enter your system from the air you breathe, the food and drink you consume, the chemicals you are exposed to, or the toxins and allergens produced by micro-organisms that inhabit your intestines.

Assess

Detox is a process that occurs naturally in your body on a continuing basis. Usually, however, it's a question of taking one step forward and one step back again, for as quickly as the toxins are removed, new ones are encountered… except when following a detox programme. The basis of detox is to reduce the amount of toxins you are exposed to so that your body can cope effectively with those already lodged in your system.

What are toxins?

A toxin is an agent that is capable of harming any body system. Toxins are classed as exogenous, endogenous or autogenous. Exogenous toxins come from external sources, e.g. tobacco, drugs, stimulants, amalgam fillings, exhaust fumes, carbon monoxide, lead, nitrogen dioxide and sulphur dioxide. Emotional factors such as stress, anxiety, grief and depression are also included in this category.

Endogenous toxins result from viral or bacterial infections, and the by-products of the metabolism of certain bacteria and yeasts that inhabit the bowel. Autogenous toxins are generated by the body itself as a result of its metabolism.

Do you need to detox?

If you are considering following a detox programme, you have probably noticed a variety of non-specific symptoms that you suspect are due to toxic overload. These could include some of the following:

Symptoms of Toxicity
✧   Flushing
✧   Palpitations
✧   Rapid pulse
✧   Dizziness
✧   Faintness
✧   Cramps

- ✧ Pins and needles
- ✧ Insomnia, disturbed sleep or unrefreshing sleep
- ✧ Drowsiness
- ✧ Physical tiredness, exhaustion, lethargy or fatigue
- ✧ Headache
- ✧ Indigestion, heartburn or peptic ulcers
- ✧ Loss of appetite
- ✧ Food cravings
- ✧ Food allergies
- ✧ Nausea
- ✧ Bloating
- ✧ Swollen ankles due to fluid retention
- ✧ Flatulence
- ✧ Diarrhoea
- ✧ Constipation
- ✧ Haemorrhoids
- ✧ Frequency of urination
- ✧ Recurrent infections
- ✧ Allergic conditions (including eczema, hives, asthma)
- ✧ Excess mucus (nose, ears, throat or stools)
- ✧ Sinus congestion
- ✧ Halitosis (bad breath)
- ✧ Inflammatory conditions, including gout, joint pains, psoriasis
- ✧ Acne, spots, pimples, boils
- ✧ Profuse sweating
- ✧ Premenstrual syndrome
- ✧ Cough
- ✧ Wheeziness
- ✧ Sore throat
- ✧ Tight or stiff neck
- ✧ Poor circulation to parts of the body
- ✧ Raised blood fat levels
- ✧ Backache
- ✧ Dry, itchy skin
- ✧ Cellulite (orange-peel skin)
- ✧ Recurrent itchy or inflamed eyes
- ✧ Waking with puffy eyes or dark circles underneath them
- ✧ Fluctuating weight, excess weight or obesity
- ✧ Low sex drive
- ✧ Difficulty conceiving

Place a tick against any of the listed symptoms that you

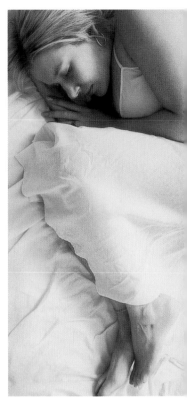

suffer from regularly: the more you have ticked, the more likely you are to need a detox. Bear in mind, however, that you should always tell your doctor about any recurrent symptoms that worry you, as they could indicate a more serious medical condition that needs further investigation or treatment.

Toxic Habits to Avoid

The old saying that "You are what you eat" is increasingly recognized as true. People following a healthy, organic, whole-food diet with a good intake of vitamins, minerals, antioxidants and protective phytochemicals, which are substances found in plants that have a beneficial effect in the human body are less likely to have long-term health problems than those eating a poor diet of processed foods and take-aways containing excess fat, salt, sugar and additives. The more of the following dietary pointers you tick, the more likely you are to benefit from a detox programme:

- ✧ Eating a mainly non-organic diet
- ✧ Regularly drinking unfiltered tap water
- ✧ Regularly drinking tea, coffee or other caffeinated beverages
- ✧ Regularly using artificial sweeteners
- ✧ Regularly eating fried foods
- ✧ Regularly eating convenience or fast foods
- ✧ Regularly eating processed foods (e.g. white rice, white bread) rather than wholefoods (e.g. brown rice, wholemeal bread)
- ✧ Adding salt to food when cooking and at the table
- ✧ Regularly eating salted foods (e.g. salted peanuts, olives, foods canned in brine)

- Regularly eating smoked foods (e.g. smoked kippers, salmon, bacon, cheese)
- Regularly eating sugar or confectionery (sweets, chocolates etc.)
- Regularly eating barbecued, char-grilled or processed meats
- Using aluminium cookware (which should be replaced as aluminium can leach into foods and build up in the body to produce toxic effects)

Toxic Habits to Give Up

A number of lifestyle and personal factors can also indicate that you need to detox. These include:

- Drinking more than two alcoholic drinks per day
- Smoking
- Using illegal drugs
- Working long hours with no time for relaxation or pleasurable activities
- Absenteeism
- Having mercury amalgam fillings in your mouth
- Taking painkillers regularly
- Undergoing a recent course of antibiotics

Again, the more factors you tick, the more likely you are to benefit from detox.

Is Your Environment Toxic?

Exposure to environmental toxins can also take their toll on your overall health. Tick any of the following factors that apply to you:

- Living near an industrial site with exposure to industrial fumes
- Living near a main road with exposure to traffic fumes
- Living in the country with exposure to farm chemicals, such as fertilizers and pesticides
- Living near high-voltage power cables
- Living near a major airport or flight path
- Working in an industry where toxic chemical exposure occurs (e.g. paints, solvents, heavy metals)
- Working in a town or city with exposure to traffic and industrial fumes
- Exposure to electromagnetic pollution from x-rays, microwaves and ultraviolet radiation
- Exposure to fumes from leaking gas appliances in the home (use kits to check regularly for carbon monoxide leaks)

Toxicity and Stress

Some emotional symptoms have also been linked with excess toxins. Those that might indicate a need to detoxify your life and to reduce your stress levels include the following:

- Uneasiness
- Tension
- Loss of sense of humour
- Difficulty concentrating
- General feeling of dullness
- Poor memory
- Forgetfulness
- Negative self-talk
- Mental tiredness
- Mood swings
- Depression
- Irritability
- Angry outbursts
- Overwhelming feelings of anxiety and panic

It is important that you detox when your body tells you it is time to do so. I see a lot of people who succumb to popular fashion in starting a cleansing programme, and who end up having a miserable experience with few positive results. If you listen, your body will let you know when it is ready.

When should I start a detox programme?

Spring is traditionally seen as the ideal time to embark on a detox programme. Another popular time is in January, following the excesses of Christmas and the pressure of New Year resolutions.

Once adhering to a detoxified lifestyle, many people choose to follow a juice fast for one day a week, for a few consecutive days each month, or for a week once or twice a year to give their body a regular detox boost.

How long does it take?

Unfortunately, detox has to go at its own pace – it can't be speeded up. Just about every cell in your body is renewed during the course of a year, so in theory it will take at least a year for all the toxins accumulated during your life to be mobilized and eliminated. During this time, new toxins will be encountered, and these will also need to be processed.

While you can follow a strict detox plan for a few weeks to help kick-start the process, detox should ideally be regarded more as a way of life so that you minimize the toxins you are exposed to long term.

Detox advantages
Tick any of the following benefits of detox that appeal to you:

- ✧ To cleanse and purify the body
- ✧ To rejuvenate
- ✧ To increase energy levels
- ✧ To increase feelings of vitality
- ✧ To boost your immunity
- ✧ To clarify your skin
- ✧ To improve flexibility
- ✧ To improve fertility
- ✧ To increase creativity
- ✧ To improve productivity
- ✧ To improve memory and concentration
- ✧ To lose weight
- ✧ To lower blood pressure
- ✧ To lower blood fat levels
- ✧ To improve intestinal health
- ✧ To enhance the senses so that you enjoy brighter lights, louder sounds, more intense smells and colours

Who should not detox?
Do not follow a detox programme if you are:
- Pregnant
- Breast-feeding
- Convalescing
- Receiving medical treatment (unless your doctor agrees that you are fit enough to do so)

Assessing detox needs with complementary therapies

Complementary therapies have a holistic approach based on the idea that physical health stems from emotional balance. A number of these therapies, including iridology, kinesiology, Kirlian photography and reflexology, can detect a build up of toxins in the body, and help you to decide whether or not you need to follow a detox programme.

Choosing a complementary practitioner
When choosing a practitioner of complementary medicine, bear in mind that standards of training and experience vary widely. Where possible:

- Select a therapist on the basis of personal recommendation from a satisfied client whose opinion you trust.
- Check what qualifications the therapist has, and whether he or she is registered with the relevant governing body for that therapy. You should be able find out what training has been undertaken and the code of ethics members should adhere to. The body will also be able to send you a list of qualified practitioners in your area.
- Find out how long your course of treatment will last and how much it is likely to cost.
- Ask how much experience the therapist has with detox and what the success rate is for your particular problems.

Iridology
Toxicity can be recognized through changes in the eyes, and iridology (the study of the iris) is a long-established way of doing this. The iris is as unique to the individual as a fingerprint, and each part of it relates to a particular area of the body. The eye is studied under magnification, allowing inherited genetic strengths and weaknesses to be detected, along with tendencies towards acidity, excess mucus and toxin deposits, plus dysfunctions of the major organs and systems.

The iris is made up of connective tissues containing approximately 28,000 nerve endings, all of which are connected to the brain. These allow the brain to receive continual information regarding organ functions, and the messages it receives are recorded in iris markings. Some genetic markings, such as liver deposits (known as 'psora'), are inherited and provide a blueprint of the constitution. They can often suggest weakness several years before symptoms develop. There are three constitutional types:

✧ Lymphatic: blue, blue-green, blue green-yellow, grey eyes
✧ Haematogenic: dark brown eyes
✧ Mixed biliary: hazel, light brown eyes

An experienced iridologist can detect toxicity and how heavy it is, plus the presence of metal deposits, excess acidity, congestion, or build ups of sulphur, sodium or cholesterol. Particular attention is paid to signs of the organs of elimination: the liver, skin, kidneys, bladder, lungs and lymphatic system. Iridologists also look for the presence of nerve rings, which indicate excess tension and stress. By following a cleansing and balancing detox programme, the colour of the irises will change as health improves. It usually takes years for this to occur, but sometimes iris colour becomes lighter and brighter after only a few months of following a healthier diet and lifestyle.

Kinesiology

Kinesiology is a diagnostic approach based on the idea that muscle groups are related to internal organs, glands and the circulation. Kinesiologists believe that the way muscles and reflexes respond to gentle pressure pinpoints imbalances in body function and energy flow. Food allergies are diagnosed by assessing muscle resistance when, for example, a particular food is held against the jaw or placed under the tongue. Fingertip massage of pressure points is also used to stimulate the circulation and correct any imbalances.

Kinesiologists believe that their simple tests take the guesswork out of diagnosing toxicity-related problems, as the body itself reveals what needs to be done to avoid a variety of symptoms. When diagnosis is complete, therapists offer nutritional advice, perhaps by determining which minerals and vitamins are lacking, and suggest lifestyle changes from which the body will benefit. For optimum health, four clearly defined areas are assessed:

✧ Mental/emotional balance
✧ Biochemical and nutritional balance
✧ Structural and postural balance
✧ Energy or life-force balance

Kinesiological balancing can gently remove energy blocks and release your natural zest for life through the detox process and beyond.

Kirlian photography

In this diagnostic technique the body's electromagnetic field is photographed and analysed using a Kirlian image. This is achieved by placing part of the body – usually the hands and/or feet – on a photographic plate emitting a high-voltage, high-frequency electric signal. The way the body's energy interacts with this electric signal produces an interference pattern which can be photographed to produce your own, individual electromagnetic aura, which will vary from time to time depending on your health. The patterns produced by Kirlian photography can be analysed to show which areas of your body are most affected by toxicity, and to monitor the progress of your detox programme. [NB Images made for the general public are usually black and white as colour Kirlian is expensive.]

Reflexology

The ancient art of reflexology is a diagnostic technique based on the principle that points on the hands and feet – known as reflexes – are indirectly related to all other organs, structures and functions of the body. These areas are mapped out on the hands and feet, with right corresponding to right and left to left. Applying pressure to reflex points reveals areas of tenderness, which help to pinpoint parts of the body that are especially affected by toxicity. Massaging these tender spots with tiny pressure movements is thought to stimulate nerves into sending messages to distant organs and relieving symptoms. Reflexology can improve circulation, normalize body functions and relieve a variety of toxicity-related symptoms, including migraine, mucus congestion, digestive problems and stress.

Once you have assessed your need for detox, you can start your cleansing and balancing programme.

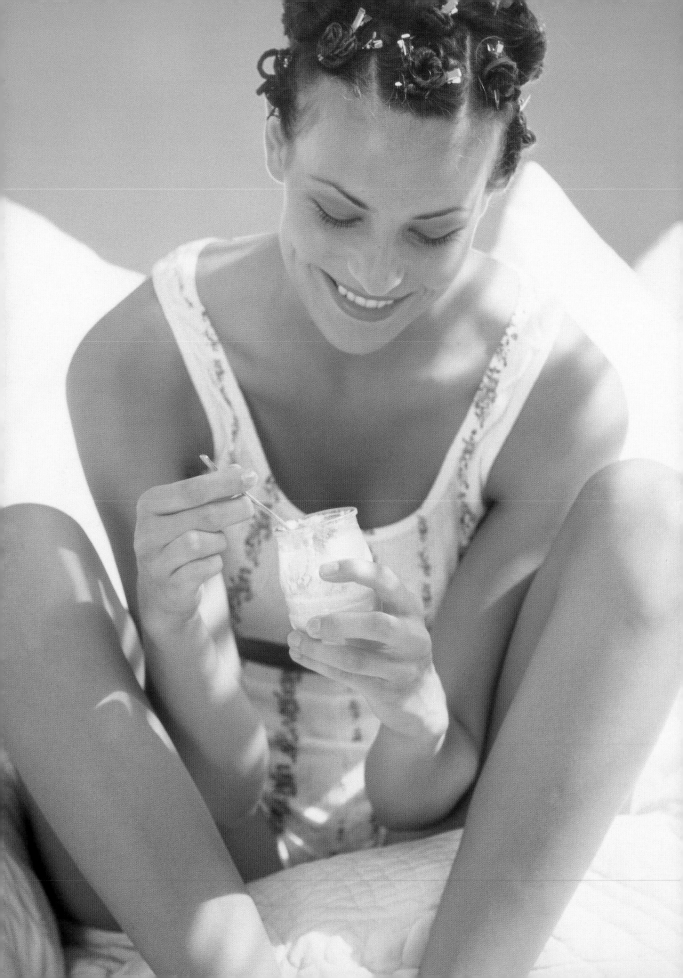

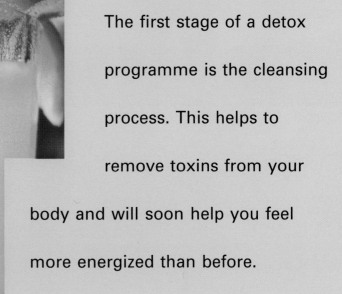

The first stage of a detox programme is the cleansing process. This helps to remove toxins from your body and will soon help you feel more energized than before.

CHAPTER THREE

Cleanse

The main aim of detox is to cleanse your body of as many toxins as possible. To do this, you need to encourage the removal of toxins already in your system and to reduce the level of new toxins you take in. The steps that will help you to cleanse your system are:

✦ juice fasting

✦ following a simple, light cleansing diet

✦ drinking plenty of fluids to flush water-soluble toxins through your kidneys

✦ going organic

✦ reducing your exposure to a variety of potentially harmful dietary and lifestyle factors, including salt, sugar, caffeine, alcohol and tobacco smoke (active and passive smoking)

✦ promoting good intestinal health through probiotic supplements

✦ supporting liver function through herbal supplements

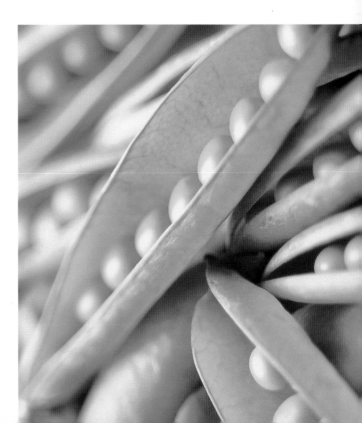

Cleaning up

Toxins are cleansed from the body in many ways, but mainly through the:

- liver – for final elimination via the lungs, kidneys and intestinal tract
- lungs – which exhale poisonous CO_2 and other gaseous/volatile waste products
- kidneys – which eliminate urea and other water-soluble toxins
- intestinal tract – which eliminates both water and fat-soluble toxins plus dietary wastes
- skin – which eliminates both water and fat-soluble waste products through evaporation, perspiration and oils (sebum)
- hair and nails – which eliminate some toxic substances, including heavy metals
- minor amounts of toxins can also be eliminated through the tears, nasal secretions, phlegm, ear wax and menstrual flow

Water-soluble toxins are mainly excreted through the urine, skin or lungs, and fat-soluble molecules are eliminated via the bile and intestinal tract.

The Liver

Weighing just over 1 kg (2.2 lb), the liver is the largest gland in the body. It lies above and largely to the right of the stomach, and has a number of important functions, including:

- making bile for digesting food
- removing environmental toxins (e.g. pesticides, fertilizers and alcohol) from the blood and inactivating them
- removing toxins produced during metabolism (e.g. ammonia formed from the metabolism of amino acids) and repackaging them into safer chemicals for excretion (e.g. urea)
- breaking down fats, hormones and excess proteins
- making glucose when needed to maintain blood sugar levels
- producing heat to warm the blood that passes through it

- making blood proteins, including those needed for blood clotting
- controlling the formation and destruction of blood cells, and recycling the iron from the red blood pigment, haemoglobin
- storage of fat-soluble vitamins (A, D, E and K) and some minerals (e.g. iron and copper)

Bile

Bile is a yellow-green fluid made in the liver, and is stored in the gall bladder until needed. When food leaves the stomach and enters the next part of the intestinal tract (the duodenum), a reflex contraction is triggered in the gall bladder, causing it to squirt bile into the duodenum, where it mixes with food. Bile contains salts and acids that break down fat globules into smaller particles, enabling them to be absorbed more easily. This process is known as emulsification.

Liver cells contain more detoxifying enzymes than any other tissues in the body as most detoxification processes start in the liver. Everything you eat or drink – with the exception of some tiny fat particles – is absorbed from the intestines and carried straight to the liver in the hepatic portal vein. The exceptions enter the lymphatic system instead.

The liver cleanses toxins from the body by transforming fat-soluble chemicals into water-soluble compounds so that they can be eliminated from the body through the bowels, kidneys, lungs and sweat. It generally detoxifies drugs, environmental toxins and cancer-causing agents by conjugating (joining) them with other chemical substances. Combining the toxins with these substances makes them more soluble and easier to eliminate from the body. This conjugation process is carried out by a family of detoxification enzymes.

Some of the chemicals produced during the first stage of liver detoxification are even more toxic than the original toxin (acetaldehyde, for example, is more toxic than alcohol). These super-toxins are then conjugated with other substances that tend to make them less toxic, and also water soluble so that they can be eliminated more easily from the body.

If the second-stage reactions are inefficient or overwhelmed by excessive production of intermediate toxins during the first stage, these super-toxins can build up in the body to trigger a so-called toxic detox (see page 24). However, supplements can be taken to help reduce the side effects of super-toxins, and to boost the activity of the second phase of liver detox reactions (see page 39).

Long-term exposure to particular toxins, such as alcohol or 3-hydroxybenzopyrene found in tobacco smoke, increases production of the detox enzymes needed to process them, so the body becomes increasingly resistant to that particular toxin. This means that when you start a detox programme, the toxins to which you have been most exposed are cleared most efficiently from your body.

Below: *The air we breathe is not always the purest so our lungs are essential to the process of filtering out toxins*

Liver Detox Mechanisms

The liver clears toxins from the body in three main ways:

- by chemically altering it and making it water soluble so that it is more easily eliminated through the kidneys
- by secreting it into bile so it is likely to pass out of the body through the intestines
- by phagocytosis, a process in which certain liver cells engulf and digest toxins, bacteria and viruses

The Lungs

The two lungs bring blood from the circulation and inspired air into close contact through their 2,400 km (1,440 miles) of airways, which provide a total surface area of 180 sq m (216 sq yd). Once air reaches the lungs, it enters the 700 million tiny air spaces known as alveoli. The alveoli are surrounded by a network of fine blood vessels called capillaries. Gaseous exchange occurs through the thin walls of the alveoli, so oxygen passes from the air sacs into the capillaries and binds with haemoglobin in red blood cells. The poisonous cell waste gas, carbon dioxide, passes in the other direction – from the blood to the alveoli – for excretion. Volatile toxins such as acetone are also excreted through the lungs. Every minute, around 6 litres (10 ½ pints) of air is breathed in, and a similar volume exhaled. This makes the lungs an efficient elimination system for gaseous/volatile toxins.

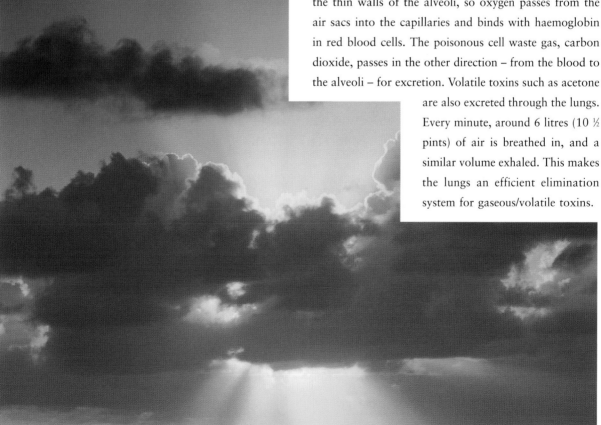

The Kidneys

The two kidneys are bean-shaped organs at the back of the abdomen. They regulate body fluid and salt levels, control blood acidity and filter out water-soluble toxins from the circulation. The kidneys contain over a million filtration units, known as nephrons. Blood flows into the tiny blood vessels of the filtration units under pressure, forcing fluid and soluble substances, such as urea (made in the liver as a by-product of protein metabolism), across the capillary walls. The filtered fluid and toxins are then concentrated as nutrients, and some water and salts are re-absorbed back into the circulation. The remaining wastes are then voided as urine. The kidneys filter up to 7 litres (12 pints) of fluid from blood every hour, making them an efficient means of cleansing water-soluble toxins from the body.

The Intestinal Tract

Swallowed food – including dietary toxins – passes into the stomach for digestion. The stomach is the most elastic part of the body and can stretch to hold 2 litres (3 ½ pints) of fluid. The stomach wall contains glands that secrete hydrochloric acid and powerful enzymes to break down complex food molecules into simpler chemicals. Gastric glands produce around 3 litres (5 pints) of acidic secretions per day. Food spends around six hours in the stomach. Muscles in the stomach wall produce a churning motion that breaks food up into smaller particles to form a semi-digested, creamy slurry known as chyme. Wave-like muscle contractions push chyme downwards through the exit from the stomach (pyloric sphincter) into the small intestines from time to time. Here, conditions are alkaline because of fluids secreted by the duodenal walls and pancreas gland. It is at this stage of digestion that bile from the liver is squirted into the chyme to emulsify fats into smaller particles for absorption. The walls of the small intestines are covered in tiny projections called villi. These absorb nutrients and toxins from the bowel into blood capillaries to take them directly to the liver. Some small globules of fat are also absorbed into the lymphatics. Dietary wastes – mostly consisting of fibre – provide

bulk to propel intestinal contents on to the large bowel. Here, bacterial fermentation breaks down some fibre, while excess water is absorbed to solidify waste remains. Probiotic supplements line the intestines with friendly bacteria, which help to maintain a healthy intestinal tract and reduce the number of toxin-producing harmful microbes. The liver secretes some toxins into the bile for elimination through the intestinal tract. Dietary fibre acts like a sponge, absorbing these toxins and preventing their re-absorption, thus assisting in their elimination.

The Skin

With a surface area of up to 2 sq m (21 sq ft), the skin forms the largest organ in the body. It has several important functions, which include providing a waterproof barrier that protects against physical damage and infection, helping to control body temperature, and making vitamin D on exposure to sunlight. It is also an important elimination organ, containing sweat glands that can excrete water-soluble toxins, and oil glands that can eliminate some fat-soluble toxins. It also eliminates toxins through the process of sloughing off dead skin.

In most places, skin is around 2mm (1/10 in) thick and is made up of two layers: an outer epidermis and an inner dermis. As newly formed cells move from the basal layer of the dermis towards the surface, they gradually become flattened and hardened, and die to produce a tough,

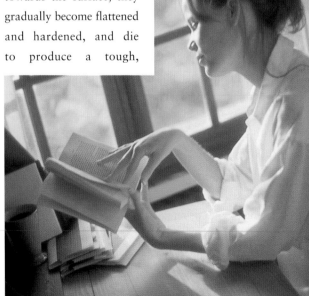

Right: *Relax and enjoy your detox programme as you feel your health improve*

water-proof outer layer for the body that is continually worn away and replaced. The body sheds 18 kg (40 lb) of skin cells during an average lifetime, and is the main contributor to household dust.

Skin brushing encourages the removal of dead cells, as well as stimulating the circulation, which assists the removal of further toxins through the sweat and oil glands. It also helps to open the pores so that the skin can breathe. Brush skin daily with a natural, vegetable bristly skin brush, using a softer brush on the face. Skin is brushed dry – do not use water – and bathe afterwards in a warm (not hot) bath or shower. You will experience a wonderful afterglow and softer, lovelier skin will result.

Wear loose clothes made from natural fibres, such as cotton or silk, next to the skin. Synthetic materials are not usually as absorbent as natural fibres and may contain coal tar products that can irritate the skin.

During detox, try to avoid using cosmetic powders, creams or oils, except for those based on evening primrose oil. If you can't do without cosmetics, try to keep them to a minimum.

Antiperspirants

In recent times there has been scientific speculation that using underarm antiperspirants could be linked with an increased risk of breast cancer because the natural purging of toxins from the body is impeded. This is an interesting but unproven hypothesis. Inasmuch as antiperspirants, like fatty diets and high incomes, are found mainly in wealthy Western societies where various cancers are also on the increase, there could be a correlation. As yet, however, there is no firm proof and many researchers feel that underarm toxins would merely be eliminated elsewhere. Research continues, however, into the possible adverse effects of parabens – preservatives added to antiperspirants. While there is no evidence at present to suggest that we should stop using underarm products, it is perhaps worth going without them during a detox programme. In the long term you might like to avoid underarm products containing parabens.

The Hair and Nails

Hairs are tubes of keratin protein that grow from follicles in the lower layer (dermis) of the skin. Nails are plates of hard, fibrous keratin produced by active cells in the base and sides of each nail. These growing areas are protected by folds of skin called cuticles. Some metals and other toxins are eliminated from the body through the hair and nails. Indeed, hair analysis is one way of assessing mineral deficiencies and toxin exposure.

Fasting

Fasting has been practised since ancient times and is an important ritual in some religions. Many holistic practitioners believe that controlled dietary restriction is beneficial to health, as it helps to clear the body of toxins that are released when body-fat stores are burned up. Some believe that fasting helps to increase spiritual awareness, and it might even delay the ageing process by increasing the production of growth hormones.

Fasting is often described as a multi-dimensional experience in which you are affected physically, mentally, emotionally and spiritually.

Several fasting regimes are in popular use:
- ✧ Water only (at least 2 litres (3 ½ pints) mineral, spring or distilled water daily)
- ✧ Juice only (e.g. apple or carrot)
- ✧ live bio yoghurt and juice
- ✧ mono, a regime in which a single food, such as apples or grapes, is eaten, usually followed with water, although juice can be taken depending on personal preference

It is not a good idea to follow a strict fast on your own without guidance from a trained professional, such as an experienced naturopath or a doctor trained in ayurvedic medicine. The detox programme outlined in this book recommends that you follow a simple, light cleansing diet, which includes organic juice, fruit, vegetables, live bio yoghurt and cottage cheese rather than a traditional fast. If you wish, however, you can have nothing but fruit juice and live bio yoghurt for one – or at most two – days at the very beginning of the programme. This is because a fast that is too strict or prolonged is stressful for the body, and might result in a so-called toxic detox for people who have led a particularly toxic lifestyle.

Toxic detox is thought to occur when toxins are mobilized from fat stores and released into the circulation in larger amounts than can be eliminated immediately. The liver's enzyme systems become overloaded and, as a result, higher than normal levels of toxins will circulate in the bloodstream. Toxic detox is associated with feeling unwell and can trigger inflammation, skin rashes and pain in the muscles or joints. In fact, it can lead to the "feeling worse before you feel better" syndrome that many people experience when embarking on a strict, water-only fast. If you feel awful, listen to your body and stop what you are doing. You have been subjecting yourself to the stress of toxic detox and should revert to a simple cleansing diet rather than continuing to fast.

Juice Fast

If you wish to fast for a day or two, it is best to opt for a juice and yoghurt fast rather than a water-only fast, which is too harsh a regime for most people.

When fasting, some lean tissue (muscle) is inevitably broken down. This effect is reduced if some energy is supplied by drinking juices that contain glucose. Even small intakes of glucose protect muscle tissue, an effect that is known as protein-sparing.

Fasting initially stimulates the liver to convert glycogen, its starchy, storage compound, to glucose and energy. Body-fat stores also start to be raided to mobilize free fatty acids as a fuel for certain body cells. Some 90 per cent of the energy needs of brain and nerve cells normally come from glucose, although other energy sources can be used during prolonged starvation. During short-term fasts, the liver makes new glucose from certain amino acids to maintain a steady supply to the central nervous system.

Fatty acids released from body-fat stores are also used as an energy source during fasting, as they convert to chemicals known as keto acids. Some of these keto acids are also converted to potentially harmful, ketone bodies, which the liver has difficulty breaking down. As a result, they spill over into the circulation. When fasting for more than a couple of days, ketone bodies are over-produced,

and a state known as ketosis develops. During ketosis, acetone is eliminated from the body in urine and through the lungs, and its distinctive odour (like pear-drops) can be detected on the breath.

Although ketones act as an important source of energy, ketosis can be dangerous. When intakes of glucose (derived from dietary carbohydrates) are low, the ability of tissues to detox ketone bodies is rapidly exceeded, so they continue to accumulate in the circulation. This results in excess acidity (metabolic acidosis) which can be severe and even fatal. During a prolonged water-only fast, or when following a very-low-calorie diet for more than a few days, the level of ketones should be monitored to avoid the dangers of ketoacidosis. Small intakes of carbohydrate, such as sugars found in fruit juices, help to feed ketones into the enzyme pathway that breaks them down and protect against ketosis. Carbohydrates are therefore said to be anti-ketogenic.

With juice fasting, there is less ketosis and you will feel more energized than when on a water-only fast, as the simple carbohydrates provided by the juices provide glucose for cell functions. Fruit and vegetable juices are also rich sources of vitamins, minerals, antioxidants and protective detoxifying plant substances known as phytochemicals, which will get your detox plan off to a good start.

Eating live bio yoghurt, which contains friendly bacteria, also helps to maintain intestinal health while toxins are eliminated.

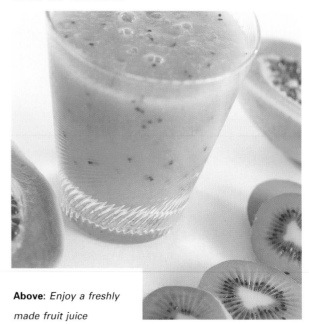

Above: *Enjoy a freshly made fruit juice*

Do not fast if you:

- are underweight
- are pregnant or breast-feeding
- are under extreme stress
- have anaemia
- have type 1 (early onset) diabetes
- are taking a prescription medication that should not be stopped
- have kidney failure
- have severe liver disease
- suffer from gout (except under specialist supervision)

Some practitioners also advise females not to fast during menstruation.

How Long Should You Fast?

If you choose to follow a fluid-only fast, this can usually be done safely for one day a week, or for two or three days on an occasional basis. Do not follow a strict fast for more than three days, except under the supervision of an experienced nutritional therapist, such as a qualified naturopath or a practitioner of ayurvedic medicine. If you suffer from a medical condition or are taking prescribed drugs, always seek medical advice first. If you start to feel awful, stop.

During a juice fast

Do not:

- take any drugs, including those bought over the counter
- smoke cigarettes
- drink caffeinated drinks
- drink alcohol
- take any supplements, except *Lactobacillus acidophilus* (a probiotic for a healthy bowel)
- take exercise, except for gentle stretching and pottering walks
- take hot baths or showers – have warm ones only

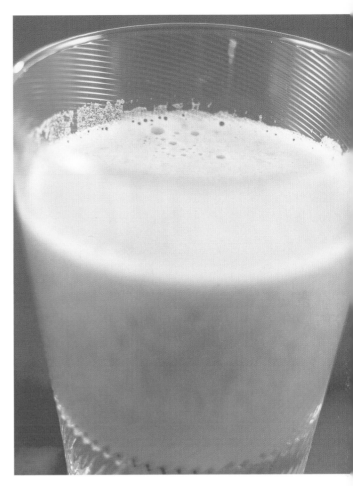

Above: *Experiment with a variety of fruits to create your own tasty juice concoctions*

Fresh Juice Detox Concoctions

When detoxing, it is best to produce your own juices from organic produce if you can. Once you've tasted freshly prepared, home-made juices, you will have little interest in those you can buy. Fresh juices have a creamy texture, a milky hue and a vastly superior taste. Their concentration also means that you can obtain significantly more vitamins and minerals than by eating raw fruit and vegetables alone. A 100-ml (3 ½-fl oz) glass of carrot juice, for example, provides as many antioxidant carotenoids as 450 g (1 lb) of raw carrots. Fresh juices also have enzyme activity, which is missing from bottled juices that have been pasteurized. Home-prepared juices can be used to make soups, but are also a great base for non-alcoholic cocktails. One of the nicest lemonades is made simply by mixing juiced lemon (plus a little peel) with sparkling mineral water and organic honey.

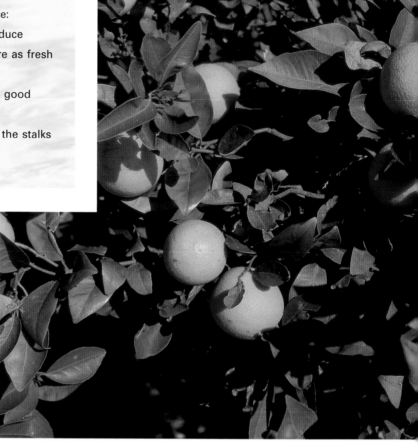

Shopping tips

When buying fruit and vegetables to juice:

- use only organic, non-waxed produce
- make sure fruit and vegetables are as fresh as possible
- choose firm, plump pieces with a good colour
- buy seedless grapes and remove the stalks to avoid bitterness

Above: *Buy fruit that is as fresh as possible to guarantee maximum benefits*

Try not to produce more juice than you need for one drinking session. Fresh juices start to deteriorate and discolour quickly (e.g. apple, kiwi fruit, avocado, carrot) and must be drunk almost immediately. Others (e.g. orange, grapefruit) can be kept chilled in the fridge for up to a day. If buying juices, select those labelled as organic, which use only vitamin C (ascorbic acid) as a preservative, and which do not have added sugar. If necessary, sweetness can be provided by organic honey.

Lemon, watermelon and apple juices have the best reputation for detox.

Fruit-based juices

(all made from fresh produce)

Juices based on apple, lemon and watermelon have excellent cleansing properties and are therefore particularly useful during detox. While juices made from one type of fruit are perfectly acceptable, you might like to try some of the following combinations for more flavour and interest. Replace apple and watermelon with lemon for additional ideas.

- Apple and banana
- Apple and blackberry
- Apple and black cherry
- Apple and blackcurrant
- Apple and fig
- Apple and lemon
- Apple and mint
- Apple and strawberry
- Grape, apricot, passion fruit and mango
- Kiwi fruit and strawberry
- Mango and apple
- Mango and orange
- Melon and passion fruit
- Melon, peach and kiwi fruit
- Melon and raspberry
- Nectarine and papaya
- Orange, avocado and strawberry
- Orange, grapefruit and lime
- Orange and strawberry
- Peach and apricot
- Pink grapefruit and pineapple
- Pink grapefruit and root ginger
- Tangerine and melon
- Watermelon and apple
- Watermelon, apple and lemon

Vegetable-based juices

(all made from fresh produce)

While juices made from one type of vegetable are perfectly acceptable, you might like to try some of the following combinations for more flavour and interest.

◇ Carrot and watercress
◇ Celery, carrot and beetroot
◇ Cucumber, beetroot and tomato
◇ Green pepper, lettuce and carrot
◇ Red pepper, carrot and parsley
◇ Red pepper, tomato and coriander
◇ Spinach, tomato and celery
◇ Tomato with black pepper
◇ Tomato, basil and garlic
◇ Tomato, celery and parsley
◇ Tomato, cucumber and spring onion

Note: Tomatoes and peppers are actually fruits, but are included here as vegetables because of their savoury flavours.

Below: Home-made juices are far superior to those you can buy

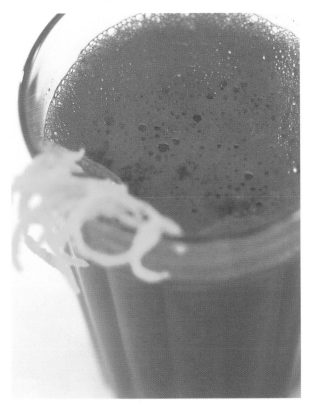

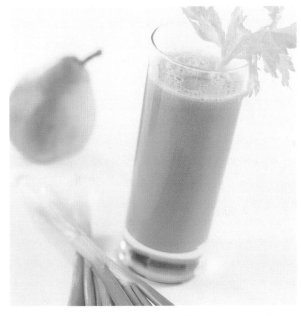

Above: *Use fruit and vegetables for different taste experiences*

Mixed fruit and vegetable juices

(all made from fresh produce)

◇ Apple and fennel
◇ Apple, celery and root ginger
◇ Apple, celery, watercress and courgette
◇ Apple, lettuce and tomato
◇ Apple, sage and spring onion
◇ Avocado, carrot and orange
◇ Carrot and lemon
◇ Carrot and orange
◇ Carrot and pear
◇ Carrot, apple and root ginger
◇ Carrot, celery and apple
◇ Carrot, pear, lettuce and parsley

Side effects of Fasting

In a water-only fast, hunger usually disappears after the first day. When on a fast that includes juices or certain foods, hunger pangs tend to continue. If you prolong a fluid-only fast for three days (or longer under supervision), you might experience some of the following side effects, which can be due to low blood glucose levels or associated with mobilized toxins. These symptoms are less likely when following a juice and yoghurt fast for one or two days before starting the cleansing diet.

Dizziness and lightheadedness

If affected, sit or lie down. Men will find it helpful to sit during urination to prevent fainting.

Palpitations

These are a common and often frightening awareness of the heartbeat, which might seem to jump, miss a beat, or be unusually strong or rapid. Palpitations normally occur after exercise and when you are under stress. They are also linked with excessive intake of caffeine, nicotine or alcohol. If palpitations occur, you should rest. If they last longer than an hour, recur over several days, or are accompanied by chest pain, shortness of breath, dizziness or faintness, contact your doctor straight away. If palpitations are associated with feelings of panic, try using Bach Rescue Remedy. Place a few drops directly under your tongue, or mix with water or juice and sip as required.

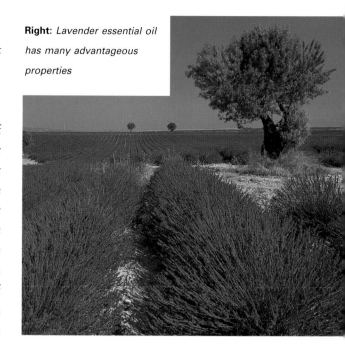

Right: *Lavender essential oil has many advantageous properties*

Headaches

One of the commonest symptoms associated with fasting, headaches can be triggered by the release of toxins and by the stress hormones produced in the body during a prolonged fast. Do not take analgesic drugs, such as aspirin, paracetamol, codeine or ibuprofen. Instead, relieve headaches with relaxation, acupressure and massage. Try getting a partner or friend to gently manipulate the muscles in your neck, shoulders and upper back.

Relieving headaches without drugs

- Try massaging the acupoint at the base of the fleshy area between your thumb and index finger – just above where the bones of these two digits meet.

- Essential oils that can help to relieve headaches include camomile, geranium, lavender, peppermint and rosemary. They may be used in all the usual ways such as diluted and massaged into the skin, inhaled and used in a diffuser. (Do not use rosemary if you have high blood pressure, and do not use any essential oils if you are pregnant.)

Insomnia

Hunger has an alerting response and it is common to find sleeping difficult during detox. To help you sleep, use relaxation exercises, visualization and – if you have a willing partner – massage. Do not take over-the-counter medications to induce sleep. Provided you are not following a water-only fast, you will find that herbal teas containing camomile, valerian, skullcap, limeflower, hops or melissa can be soothing and help to promote sleep.

Nausea

Another common symptom of detox, especially during prolonged fasting, is nausea. It can be relieved by acupressure (see below).

Relieving nausea with acupressure

Press for five minutes over the acupoint situated in the middle front of the forearm, approximately three to four fingerbreadths above the wrist crease. Stimulate this point every two or three hours to help keep nausea at bay, and whenever sickness is felt. The same effect can be obtained by wearing travel sickness wristbands, which have studs that press on the relevant points. These are available from chemists.

Bad taste in the mouth

A coated tongue and bad taste in the mouth often occur during detox, especially in the first few days of fasting. The best remedy is to scrape the tongue using a teaspoon or a plastic scraper device available from chemists, and to freshen the mouth by rinsing with diluted lemon juice.

Increased body odour

Some people notice that their body odour becomes more pronounced during detox. The obvious solution is to take daily warm (not hot) showers or baths.

Dry skin

Outbreaks of spots and dry skin can occur during detox, and are signs that you might be detoxing too fast – the so-called toxic detox. Instead of fasting, follow a simple, light cleansing diet. Moisturize using a non-perfumed body lotion – preferably one containing evening primrose oil – and use a loofah to gently exfoliate your skin in a warm bath. Adding pure evening primrose oil to your diet, will help maintain a good intake of essential fatty acids and healthy skin. Try taking gelatin-based capsules or adding drops of evening primrose oil to drinks or sprinkled on food, in dressings.

Constipation

Lack of bowel motions due to less roughage is normal when not eating solids and will occur if you choose to follow a water-only fast and sometimes occur with a juice fast or light diet. Constipation can result, as more fluid is absorbed from the bowels when transit time is slowed. People often also notice a change in colour of motions, and they may become thinner and more ribbony than usual. Taking a probiotic supplement (see page 45) will help to maintain healthy bowel flora (friendly bacteria such as lactobacilli). Taking a fibre supplement, such as psyllium husks, will help to maintain normal bowel function. When opening the bowels, avoid straining by leaning forwards at the hips.

If you choose to follow a strict water-only or juice-only fast and develop side effects that worry you, always seek medical advice. It is better and safer to follow a more gentle cleansing diet when undergoing detox because this greatly reduces the risk of side effects.

Cell refreshment

Following a detox programme gives every cell in your body the opportunity to catch up on its housekeeping functions while undergoing few new demands. This allows cells to eliminate wastes and to repair, rejuvenate and regenerate. Nowhere does this happen more spectacularly than in the liver. Even cells that have undergone fatty change and been poisoned with excess alcohol (see page 31) can eliminate this excess fat and repair themselves if alcohol is completely avoided.

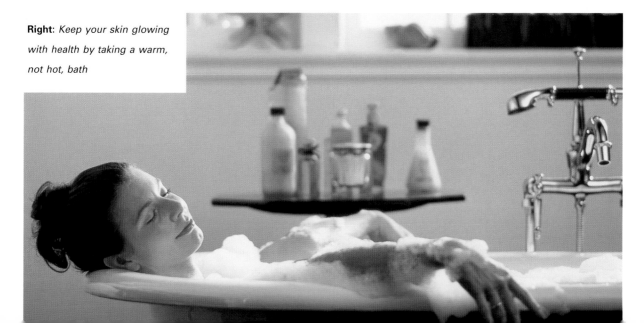

Right: *Keep your skin glowing with health by taking a warm, not hot, bath*

Light cleansing diet

If you have chosen to follow a strict fast, your stomach will have temporarily reduced in volume and the production of intestinal juices will have fallen significantly. You must therefore break a fast carefully by taking in only diluted fruit or vegetables juices, thin vegetable soups, watermelon and live bio yoghurt.

✦ If possible, all items should be organic, otherwise you are introducing more toxins into your system. Follow this light, semi-liquid diet for a day or two before starting the cleansing diet. If you have not been following a strict fast, you can start the cleansing diet straight away. This involves having nothing but filtered or mineral water with organic fruit and/or vegetable juices, thin vegetable soups, steamed vegetables, cooked pulses, oatmeal, brown rice, cottage cheese, bio yoghurt, fish and chicken.

Tip

Add fresh, young dandelion leaves to salads for their cleansing action.

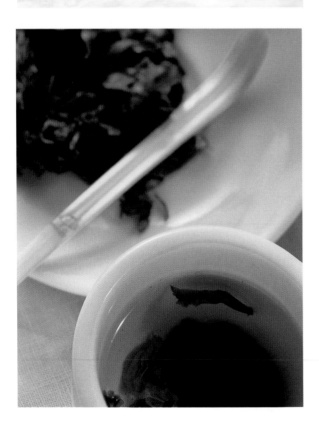

There are two important requirements of a cleansing diet. It should provide:

1. Enough energy (at least half of estimated daily needs) to reduce excess mobilization of body fats and delay the re-entry of fat-soluble toxins into the circulation.
2. Enough protein to prevent muscle wasting, while at the same time not overburdening the circulation with excess nitrogenous wastes (e.g. ammonia, urea) formed when protein is metabolized.

Suggestions on what to eat during the cleansing diet are contained in the Total Detox Plan (see page 114).

What to Avoid

The cleansing diet is as important for what it does not contain as for what it provides. Perhaps for the first time in many years, embarking on this diet means that you will not be exposing your body to excess caffeine, salt, additives, artificial sweeteners, agrochemicals (see page 33), alcohol or sugar, all of which can have a toxic effect on the body.

Caffeine

The stimulant caffeine mimics the effects of stress in the body. Drinking more than five or six caffeinated beverages per day can lead to caffeine toxicity, with symptoms of restlessness, irritability, headache, insomnia, tremor and tiredness.

During detox, it is important to cut out caffeine altogether. If you have previously had a high intake however, this can lead to withdrawal symptoms, which are similar to those of toxicity, with headache and irritability. If necessary, prepare yourself for detox by gradually cutting down on caffeinated drinks for a week or two before starting the cleansing diet. Similarly, replace every other caffeinated drink with a decaffeinated version, or with a herbal or fruit tea.
If you find it difficult to reduce your intake of caffeine, try switching to guarana (see page 82).

Salt

Table salt is commonly used to flavour food. While a certain amount is necessary for good health, excessive

Left: *Replace caffeinated beverages with herbal or fruit teas*

amounts can be toxic and have been linked with an increased risk of high blood pressure. This sensitivity depends on the genes you have inherited and affects an estimated one in two people. Even in those who are not sensitive to this effect, excess salt can cause fluid retention, bloating and make dehydration more likely.

During a detox cleansing diet, it is important not to add salt to any foods during cooking or at the table. Obtain flavour from spices, black pepper and herbs. Any

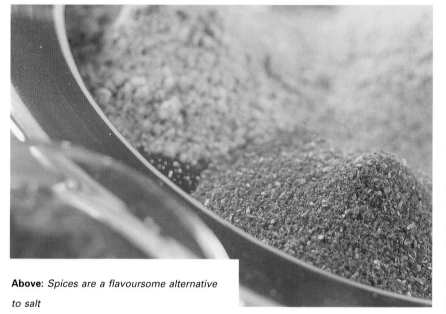

Above: *Spices are a flavoursome alternative to salt*

salt you need will be obtained naturally from the fruit and vegetables you eat, and the potassium they contain will help to flush excess salt from the body.

Try to continue the no-salt habit when reverting to a wholefood balancing diet, too. Ideally, you should take in no more than 4–6g of salt per day. By not salting food, and by avoiding all processed and precooked foods, your intake will be healthily lower than this. (Three-quarters of dietary salt is hidden in processed foods, such as ready-prepared meals, biscuits, cakes, meat products, breakfast cereals, packet soups, sauces, stock cubes and yeast extracts.)

Tip

Lime juice intensifies natural salt flavours so you miss salty flavours less. Lime juice may be sprinkled on to food or added to water and drunk with a meal.

Alcohol

Although alcohol is a powerful cell toxin, a low to moderate intake is beneficial in reducing stress and possible coronary heart disease. Alcohol is metabolized in the liver to acetaldehyde – a cellular poison – which can damage liver, brain and heart muscle cells. Long term excessive intake of alcohol is linked with four particular types of liver damage – fatty degeneration, alcoholic hepatitis, liver fibrosis and cirrhosis.

Fatty degeneration

As alcohol is such a poisonous toxin, liver cells drop their normal metabolic reactions and work overtime to eliminate alcohol from the system, converting it first into acetaldehyde (even more toxic) and then into acetate. While liver enzymes are diverted from their normal tasks, fewer fatty acids are processed or converted into the storage substance glycogen. As a result, liver cells start to accumulate unprocessed globules of fat and become abnormally swollen. Even a single episode of binge drinking can change liver cell metabolism and trigger fatty degeneration.

The impaired metabolic reactions inside liver cells generate large numbers of damaging free radicals. These increase the damaging effects of continued excessive alcohol intake, and liver cells accumulate more and more fatty globules. The liver enlarges and takes on a yellow appearance, resembling the grossly abnormal, fatty livers of the force-fed geese in France, which are used to make *pâté de foie gras*.

By this stage, the liver enzymes are seriously unbalanced. Those that break down alcohol are present in unusually large numbers. Reduced amounts of sugars and proteins are produced in the liver and a degree of malnutrition sets in. Even at this advanced stage of fatty degeneration, however, changes are reversible. Liver cells have a tremendous ability to regenerate, and following a detox programme while avoiding alcohol will, in time, help the liver to recover fully.

Alcoholic hepatitis

In some cases, a hypersensitive reaction to alcohol causes the liver to become inflamed on top of the fatty degeneration, leading to alcoholic hepatitis. This is more serious, as liver cells start to degenerate and die. Some cells accumulate a glassy-looking material, which is a protein-based substance known as amyloid, while others are converted into balls of fat. Fever, nausea and vomiting occur, with pain and tenderness over the liver area in the upper right-hand abdomen. Yellow jaundice develops as liver inflammation worsens. Recovery is followed by the formation of liver scar tissue.

Alcoholic fibrosis

A liver full of fatty degeneration will eventually lay down scar tissue (fibrosis) even if alcoholic hepatitis has not intervened. If fibrosis is extensive, it interferes with the liver's blood supply and can lead to back pressure on vessels trying to feed blood to the liver. Back pressure is pressure acting backwards, so as it builds up, it becomes increasingly difficult for blood to push forwards against it. The vessels swell, and varicose veins develop in the oesophagus, which can bleed torrentially. Fibrosis sometimes becomes progressive and leads to cirrhosis, especially if repeated attacks of alcoholic hepatitis occur.

Cirrhosis

Alcoholic cirrhosis is a serious liver disease. It develops as a result of liver cell death, fibrosis, impaired blood supply and the desperate attempt of some liver cells to regenerate new tissue. The balance between blood supply and regenerating nodules of liver is abnormal, and blood-starved cells continue to die. This triggers more fibrosis, which obliterates more blood vessels, and a vicious cycle is set up. Islands of regenerating liver cells are separated by bands of scar tissue and the liver takes on a shrunken, nobbly appearance. Owing to inadequate blood supply, these nodules of regenerated tissue fail to function properly. Back pressure on the blood supply from the gut becomes worse, and the varicose veins in the oesophagus enlarge. Alcoholic cirrhosis eventually leads to death from haemorrhage, liver failure or liver cancer. (The last develops in around 10 per cent of cases as a result of the abnormal cell regeneration.)

The more serious effects of alcohol tend to occur in people who are addicted to it. Abstinence from alcohol at this late stage can improve cirrhosis by removing the poison that is causing liver cell damage. In addition, extracts of milk thistle (see page 41) have been shown to improve liver function, even when cirrhosis is present.

During a detox programme, it is important to avoid alcohol altogether. Afterwards, limit your intake to no more than two alcoholic drinks per day and aim to have several alcohol-free days per week. The form of alcohol that, in moderation, seems most beneficial to health is red wine, mainly due to the powerful antioxidant pigments it contains. Wine should ideally be drunk with food rather than on its own, as it seems to reduce the potentially harmful effects of saturated fats through its blood-thinning action.

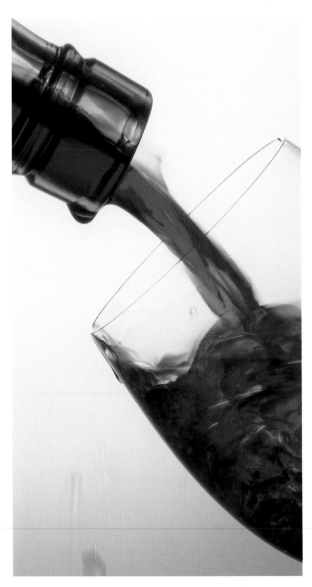

Coping with alcohol cravings
- The herb kudzu (see page 42) has helped many people, as it can dramatically decrease cravings for alcohol.
- Yerba maté tea is an energizing tonic that is also used as a substitute for alcohol. It helps liver regeneration, especially when trying to reduce alcohol intake (see page 83).
- Vitamin B5 derivatives (e.g. calcium pantothenate and pantotheine) have been found to improve liver function and boost immunity by increasing both blood levels of antibodies and the activity of white blood cells. Pantotheine produced the most pronounced therapeutic effect.

Chlorinated water

Some 80 per cent of the world's drinking water contains the bleach chlorine, which helps keep it free from bacterial infection. Impurities, such as toxic metals (lead, aluminium and cadmium), and traces of hormones have also been found in tap-water supplies and have been linked with health problems, including undescended testicles in male babies, lowered sperm counts and hormone-dependent cancers. Fitting an activated-carbon filter to your drinking water supplies can extract chlorine, while a reverse-osmosis water treatment system is needed to remove dissolved metals. Alternatively, consider drinking bottled water from a source that provides an analysis or certification of purity.

Sugar

While simple sugars are an important source of energy, they are absorbed very rapidly from the diet and can provoke potentially harmful swings in blood glucose and insulin levels. It is best to avoid simple dietary sugars, such as those provided by chocolate, and instead eat more starchy carbohydrates. These are steadily broken down during digestion into a variety of simple sugars, which are absorbed into the circulation more slowly. Changing the

Left: *Red wine may have certain benefits, but it is best to avoid all alcohol during detox*

diet in this way reduces large sugar swings and is better for health. The speed with which complex carbohydrates are broken down into simpler sugars is known as the glycaemic index (see page 57).

Artificial sweeteners

Some artificial sweeteners are increasingly being linked with toxic effects in the body. While the jury is still out on their absolute safety, they and all other artificial additives are best avoided during a cleansing and balancing detox programme.

The Fluid Flush
During detox, it is vital to drink plenty of filtered or mineral water to help flush water-soluble toxins through your kidneys and sweat glands. As a general rule, aim to drink 2–3 litres (3 ½–5 pints) of fluid per day – more if you are in a hot climate, taking exercise or sweat heavily.

Going organic

Eating and drinking organic products is essential for anyone wanting to detox. This means eating foods produced by organic farming methods and which have received minimal processing. They have not been treated with pesticides, antibiotics, hormones or artificial fertilizers, and are not the products of genetic manipulation or irradiation. Organic farmers use traditional methods of pest control and crop rotation, which result in produce that is full of flavour, vitamins and minerals, and which contains the lowest possible amounts of artificial, potentially toxic chemicals.

Non-organic crops are bred for their uniformity of colour and size and the ability to keep their appearance for longer. Often, these qualities are achieved at the expense of flavour and nutrients, and with the help of agro-chemicals, such as pesticides, weedkillers, fungicides, fumigants, growth promoters, growth retardants and fertilizers. These chemicals are applied regularly, from the time the crop is still in its seed form, during germination and throughout its growing cycle. Each non-organic apple,

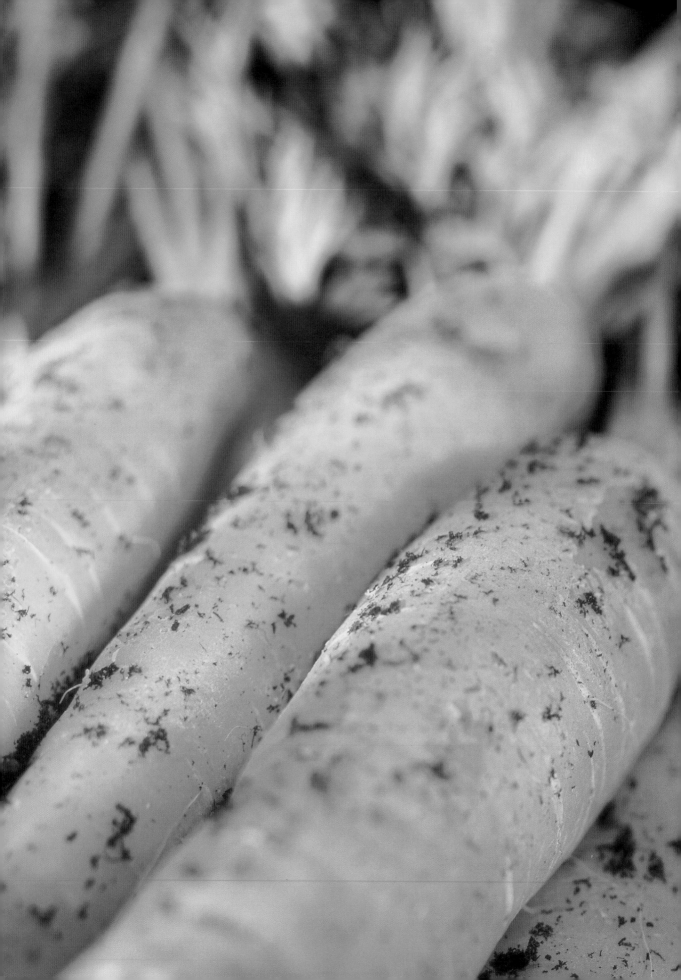

for example, has been dosed around 40 times with up to 100 additives before you eat it. These chemicals do not just lie on the surface of the produce, but are found beneath the skin and sometimes throughout the flesh itself. A lettuce is sprayed an average of 11 times in the few weeks it takes to develop. The full effects of many of these chemicals on our long-term health are still not fully understood, so it is common to hear of chemicals in widespread use one day being banned the next. The Environment Protection Agency in the United States, for example, considers that 60 per cent of all herbicides, 90 per cent of all fungicides and 30 per cent of all insecticides are potentially cancer-causing. And consuming more than one toxin at a time can greatly magnify their toxic effects.

> During the course of one year, a person following a non-organic diet consumes an estimated 6 kg (13 lb) of chemicals, including food additives, colourings, flavourings, preservatives, waxes, fertilizers, pesticides and herbicide residues.

In 1999, the Working Party on Pesticide Residues tested non-organic produce on sale in the United Kingdom. They found that:

❖ One-third of fruit and vegetables had pesticide residues – many containing four or five, and some as many as seven, different toxins

❖ 3 per cent had residues above accepted limits

❖ 100 per cent of oranges had residues – over two-thirds containing three or more different toxins

❖ 96 per cent of all pears contained residues, of which nearly half held three or more different pesticides. Some contained an illegal chemical, chlormequat, known to cause tumours in animals

❖ 84 per cent of lettuces had pesticide residues – almost half from three or more different toxins. One lettuce was found to contain a chemical that exceeded the recommended limit by over 100 times

❖ 68 per cent of apples had residues, many containing chemicals known to affect fertility

Left: *Organic produce is full of nutrients and flavour*

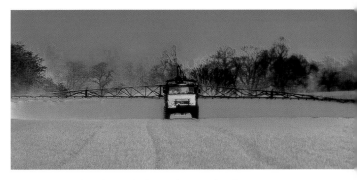

Above: *Agricultural chemicals can have toxic effects*

Organic foods

The range of organic foods available is vast and includes:

- fruit (e.g. oranges, lemons, apples, clementines, tangerines, grapefruit, grapes, pears, bananas, mangoes)
- vegetables (e.g. carrots, potatoes, onions, parsnips, courgettes, aubergines, beans, broccoli, spinach, garlic)
- salad produce (e.g. lettuce, tomatoes, cucumbers, peppers, celery, spring onions, beetroot)
- bread, rice and pasta
- milk, cream, butter and eggs
- cheeses
- meat and poultry (e.g. chicken, lamb, pork, beef, bacon)
- game (e.g. pigeon, guinea fowl, rabbit)
- fish (e.g. lemon sole, monkfish, cod, plaice, turbot, haddock, mackerel, sardines, salmon, squid, mussels, oysters, lobster, crab, etc.) caught from some of the cleanest waters in the world, which have now been declared organic
- fruit juices
- olive and nut oils
- natural spring water
- tea leaves

Almost everything you can think of is available in an organic form. Home delivery is also easy to arrange (see Soil Association, page 127).

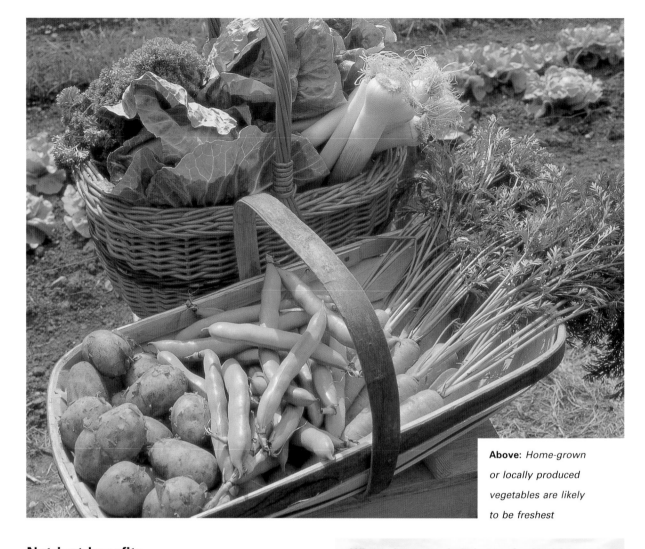

Above: *Home-grown or locally produced vegetables are likely to be freshest*

Nutrient benefits

Organic foods contain, on average, twice the vitamins, minerals, trace elements, essential fatty acids, fibre and phytochemicals in commercially grown produce. This is partly because they contain less water and more solid matter, but is also due to the rich soils in which they are grown. Non-organic crops are produced in soils boosted with artificial fertilizers that provide nitrogen, phosphorus and potassium but do not usually replenish other minerals or trace elements. In addition, crops shipped from abroad are picked before ripe, so their nutrient content is naturally low. Fresh produce that is organically grown locally and has only recently been harvested will contain the most nutrients. In the UK, organic standards are set by an EC directive. Organic foods are checked and certified by an independent body, such as the Soil Association, so you can be sure that the producers stick to a strict code of practice.

Why going organic is better for health

Chemicals used in producing or rearing non-organic foodstuffs:

- are concentrated in the liver and can lead to liver problems
- have been linked with lowered fertility
- have been associated with intestinal problems such as irritable bowel syndrome, Candida overgrowth and inflammatory bowel disease
- lower immunity and can increase the risk of allergies and certain cancers
- are linked with the emergence of resistant bacteria that are difficult to treat – it is estimated that 50 per cent of the antibiotics we consume come from meat, dairy produce since they are widely used as growth promoters

Over 50 per cent of all agro-chemicals are sprayed on fruit and vegetables to maintain their cosmetic appearance. Since organic produce is bred for flavour and nutrients rather than colour and shape, its appearance is often secondary. This is why organic fruit and vegetables might be smaller, look less attractive than standard products and contain creepy-crawlies, such as greenfly and caterpillars.

Organic produce is more attractive and vital on the inside, however, as it has not been treated with artificial, life-extending chemicals. Look for produce that is crisp and firm with a healthy colour. Reject any that look wilted, brown, faded or bruised.

Unfortunately, organic foods often cost more than their non-organic counterparts. In the long run, however, organic produce actually costs less when you consider the benefits to health. Weight for weight, they are also better value in terms of the flavour and nutrients they contain. Prices are slowly coming down as production grows to meet consumer demand. To help keep your costs down:

✧ buy fruit and vegetables in season rather than those imported at additional cost
✧ buy locally
✧ buy in bulk
✧ buy wholefoods rather than processed foods
✧ eat more plant-based foods and less meat
✧ look out for special offers
✧ join a box scheme that delivers fruit and vegetables to your door from local producers with no middle-man profit

> The organic food sector is growing at a phenomenal rate. In the UK, for example, organic production is expanding by 50 per cent a year and is expected to occupy 10 per cent of agricultural land by the year 2007.

Cleansing Supplements

A number of supplements may be taken during the cleansing phase of a detox plan. These include antioxidants, supplements to support liver function, supplements to support kidney function and supplements to support intestinal function.

Note: Do not take any supplements during a water-only fast. Take detox supplements only when following a light cleansing and balancing diet such as that described in Chapter 12. Do not take supplements during pregnancy or when breast-feeding, except under the supervision of a qualified practitioner.

Antioxidants

Antioxidants are protective substances that patrol the body, mopping up toxic by-products of metabolism. The most important

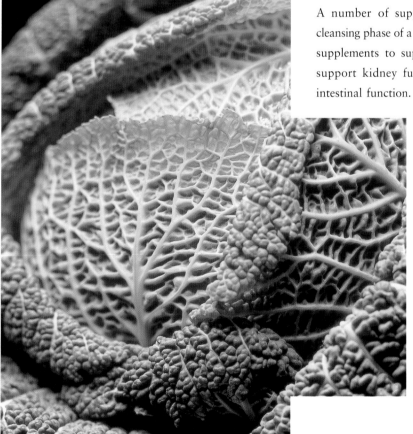

Left: *Only select crisp, firm, non-damaged produce*

dietary antioxidants are vitamin A and related carotenoids, vitamin C, vitamin E and selenium.

Antioxidants quench damaging oxidation reactions in the body. Most oxidations are triggered by free radicals – unstable molecular fragments that carry a negative electrical charge. Free radicals pass on this negative charge during collisions with other molecules and cell structures, triggering harmful chain reactions that damage proteins, fats, cell membranes and genetic material. Each body cell undergoes an estimated 10,000 free radical oxidations daily. These oxidations have been linked with hardening and furring up of the arteries, coronary heart disease, cataracts, macular degeneration of the eye, premature ageing of the skin and cancer. Free radicals are toxins generated by normal metabolic reactions as well as exposure to environmental pollutants, x-rays, ultraviolet light and some drugs. Smokers and diabetics generate more than usual.

Vitamin A

Vitamin A is a fat-soluble vitamin which can be stored in the liver. It occurs in two main forms, as pre-formed vitamin A (found in animal foods) and as carotenoids – plant pigments of which some (e.g. betacarotene) can be convertd into vitamin A in the body. Vitamin A can be toxic in excess, and most supplements therefore contain carotenes rather than vitamin A itself. Excess betacarotene (e.g. from drinking large quantities of carrot juice) causes a yellow-orange pigmentation of the skin similar to cheap fake tan. This is probably not harmful and quickly fades once intakes are reduced. It is a powerful antioxidant and is also essential for normal growth, development, sexual health and fertility. It maintains healthy skin, teeth, bones and mucous membranes such as those lining the nose, throat and eyes and is important for vision and immunity.

Sources: Vitamin A (retinol): animal and fish liver, kidneys, eggs, milk, cheese, yoghurt, butter, oily fish, meat, margarine. Foods including carotenes: sweet corn, carrots, sweet potatoes, spinach, broccoli, watercress, spring greens, mango, red/yellow peppers, tomatoes.

Dose: Supplements containing natural betacarotene (e.g. 6mg to 15mg daily) along with other fruit and vegetable extracts are available. If pure vitamin A supplements are used, they should ideally be limited to less than 5,000 IU (1,500mcg) per day (avoid during pregnancy).

Vitamin C

Being an important water-soluble antioxidant, vitamin C protects the aqueous parts of the body. In fact, so great is its importance that many animals make vitamin C themselves. Quite why man is one of the few mammals to have lost or never acquired the ability to synthesize vitamin C remains one of the greatest mysteries of human biochemistry. It is clear, however, that those with the highest intake of vitamin C have the lowest risk of developing coronary heart disease and certain cancers.

Sources: Blackcurrants, guavas, kiwi fruit, citrus fruit, mangoes, green peppers, strawberries, green-sprouting vegetables, e.g. broccoli, Brussel sprouts, watercress, parsley.

Dose: 1g three times a day (or 3g slow-release formulation once a day) during detox, and preferably in the form known as Ester-C. This contains predigested vitamin C that contains the body-ready breakdown products of vitamin C that have all the activity of the parent substance without the acidity as it has a neutral pH. As a bonus, Ester-C is absorbed into cells more quickly and stays in the body longer than standard vitamin C.

Vitamin E

Vitamin E is a powerful antioxidant that protects body fats from the toxic effects of free radicals. It also protects cell membranes, nerve sheaths, circulating cholesterol molecules, dietary fats and body fat stores from chemical attack due to free radicals. It is such a good detoxifying agent that those with the highest intakes of vitamin E have the lowest risks of developing coronary heart disease and certain cancers.

Sources: Wheatgerm oil, avocados, eggs, butter, wholemeal cereals, seeds, nuts, oily fish, broccoli.

Dose: 268 mg (400 IU) per day during detox.

Selenium

Selenium is a mineral that is needed for the action of many antioxidant enzymes, including one (glutathione peroxidase) which removes toxic substances such as hydrogen peroxide generated in the body by free radicals. As an antioxidant, selenium protects against a wide variety of degenerative diseases, such as hardening and furring of the arteries, emphysema, liver problems, cataracts, arthritis, stroke and heart attack. Trials have also shown that taking selenium daily halves the risk of death from cancer. Selenium supplements given to animals significantly improved health and prolonged life; whether or not they can do the same for humans remains to be seen. An on-going trial is looking at the effects of selenium supplements on cancer risk in over 40,000 participants in five countries (Denmark, Finland,

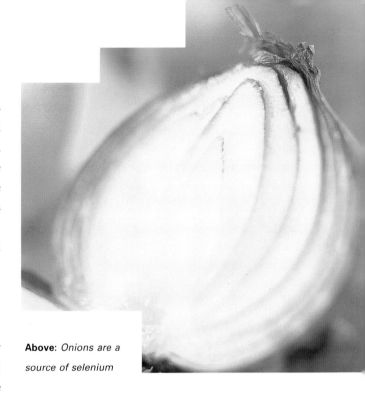

Above: *Onions are a source of selenium*

Sweden, the United Kingdom and the United States). Volunteers are randomized to receive a daily 100 mcg, 200 mcg or 300 mcg of selenium or an inactive placebo. The results after five years are expected to influence public health guidelines on optimal selenium intake for cancer prevention worldwide.

Sources: Brazil nuts, broccoli, mushrooms, cabbage, radishes, onions, garlic, celery, wholegrains, seafood.

Dose: 200 mcg per day during detox.

A variety of other antioxidant supplements are also available from natural sources, such as grapeseed, oregano and pine bark extracts. These might be individually recommended during detox if you are following a programme overseen by a naturopathic practitioner.

Supplements to Support Liver Function

A number of traditional herbal remedies are able to cleanse and support liver function, including dandelion, globe artichoke, gotu kola, milk thistle, sarsaparilla, turmeric and kudzu.

Artichoke extracts (Cynara scolymus)

Globe artichoke is a perennial, culinary plant cultivated for its large heads containing fleshy scales with an edible

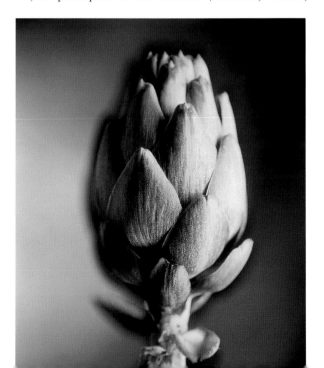

Left: *Globe artichoke leaves are used to support liver function*

base. Extracts of globe artichoke leaves contain unique compounds, such as cynarin, which have liver-regenerating effects similar to those of the milk thistle. Cynara also stimulates bile production and can quickly relieve symptoms of nausea, bloating and indigestion caused by insufficient bile production. In a randomized, double-blind, placebo-controlled trial, artichoke extracts were shown to increase bile production by over 127 per cent within 30 minutes, and by over 150 per cent after 60 minutes. No side effects were reported.

Dose: 300–600 mg of standardized extracts per day (the equivalent to 16 g/½ oz of fresh leaves) during detox.

Dandelion (Taraxacum officinalis)

Dandelion is a well-known perennial weed found in most parts of the world. The leaves were traditionally eaten in spring as a cleansing herbal tonic. Dandelion root (usually obtained from two-year-old plants) also has an important

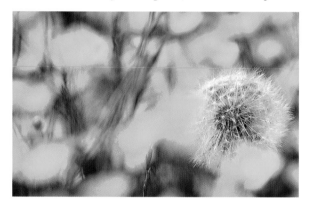

Above: *Extracts from the dandelion can support liver and kidney function*

cleansing action that is widely used during detox programmes. It promotes the steady elimination of toxins through a variety of routes. On the liver, it increases detoxification functions and stimulates the flow of bile so that more toxins are eliminated through the bowels. On the kidneys, it has a diuretic action that increases the elimination of water-soluble toxins from the body. It also has a gentle laxative action to promote the elimination of toxins through the bowels. In addition, dandelion contains useful minerals, including potassium, which helps to flush out excess sodium.

Dose: 5–10 g per day in three divided doses. Do not use if you have gallstones.

Garlic (Allium sativum)

Thanks to its popularity in cooking, garlic has a worldwide average consumption equivalent to one clove per person per day. Long known to be antiseptic, antibacterial and antiviral, it is used to treat stomach and respiratory infections. It also contains a number of substances that promote the action of key liver detoxification enzymes and has a beneficial effect on circulating blood-fat levels. Clinical trials using standardized garlic powder tablets have shown that regular garlic consumption can reduce high blood pressure, lower levels of harmful blood fats (LDL-cholesterol and triglycerides), reduce blood stickiness and improve circulation to all parts

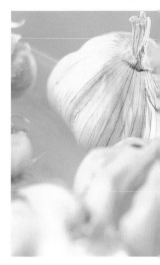

Above: *Garlic can lower blood fat levels*

of the body. Regular use reduces the risk of hardening and furring of the arteries by up to 25 per cent, and the risk of a heart attack by up to 50 per cent. Garlic has also been shown to support desirable bowel bacteria, such as lactobacilli, and to inhibit undesirable microbial flora.

Dose: 600–900 mg standardized garlic powder tablets per day.

Note that garlic products made by solvent extraction or by boiling garlic in oil seem to be less effective than tablets made from freeze-dried and powdered garlic.

Gotu kola (Centella asiatica)

A herbaceous perennial creeper native to India, China, Indonesia, Australia, the South Pacific, Madagascar and parts of Africa, gotu kola is reputed to increase longevity, hence its alternative name – the fountain of youth. Legend claims that gotu kola was used by a Chinese herbalist called Li-Ching Yun, who reputedly lived to the age of 256. In Asia, many people regularly eat one leaf of the plant a day in the hope of prolonging life. Gotu kola is not related to the kola nut and does not contain caffeine.

Regarded as one of the most important herbs in ayurvedic medicine, brahmi, as it is also known, is used to relieve anxiety and depression, improve memory, promote calmness, relax muscle tension, boost adrenal function during times of stress and relieve pain. It is also said to have blood-cleansing properties and to increase physical and mental energy levels. In patients with liver cirrhosis, Centella has been shown to improve the microscopic appearance of liver tissue and to reduce inflammation. The active ingredients are known as triterpenes.

Dose: 2–4 capsules per day of standardized extracts containing 25 mg triterpenes. High doses, which might cause headaches, are calming rather than energizing.

Milk Thistle
(Silybum marianum or Carduus marianus)

A thorny, weed-like plant with purple flower-heads, milk thistle is native to Mediterranean Europe. Its seeds contain a powerful mixture of antioxidants known as silymarin, of which the most active ingredient is silibinin. Historically, milk thistle heads were boiled and eaten like globe artichokes as a spring tonic to protect the liver.

More than 300 studies have shown that silymarin can protect liver cells from the poisonous effects of excess alcohol and other toxins, such as those produced by the death cap mushroom and chemotherapy. It works by inhibiting factors responsible for liver cell damage – e.g. free radicals – and by maintaining levels of an important liver antioxidant enzyme called glutathione. Silymarin also seems to alter the outer structure of liver cell walls so that poisons do not penetrate as readily. In addition, silymarin stimulates protein synthesis of the liver cells, which helps the liver regenerate itself after damage, such as that caused by fibrosis. It has recently been shown to have a protective effect on kidney cells as well. Silymarin also inhibits depletion of one of the liver's most important antioxidant enzymes, glutathione, which is needed to break down alcohol and other liver toxins. As an antioxidant, silymarin is at least 200 times more potent than vitamins C or E, and is being investigated as a possible protective agent against ultraviolet-induced skin cancers.

Dose: Standardized supplements of 70–200 mg three times per day.

It is best to start with a low dose and slowly increase. Liver function will start to show an improvement within five days and continue over at least the next three weeks.

The only reported side effect is mild bowel stimulation in some people due to increased production of bile.

Sarsaparilla (Smilax officinalis)

This climbing perennial vine contains a wide range of hormone-like substances. It is used mainly as a blood purifier, believed to bind bacterial toxins and cholesterol in the gut so that lower amounts are absorbed into the circulation, and reducing the workload of the liver and other organs. It also acts as a diuretic and promotes sweating and expectoration of catarrh. The best sarsaparilla is said to produce a slightly nauseating, acrid taste in the mouth, and even to cause a burning sensation. In some people it can cause indigestion, and if taken to excess, can temporarily impair kidney function. Some practitioners advise against its use in women prone to excessive superfluous hair.

Dose: 250 mg capsules three times per day.

Turmeric (Curcuma longa)

Turmeric is an orange-yellow spicy root widely used in Asian cooking. It is also a traditional ayurvedic and Chinese herbal medicine used for treating liver problems, such as jaundice and bloating. Turmeric contains an anti-inflammatory antioxidant, curcumin, that stimulates secretion of bile and boosts liver function by increasing levels of antioxidant enzymes

Above: *Turmeric contains the antioxidant curcumin*

in the liver. It also supports liver regeneration, reduces blood-clotting and helps to lower raised cholesterol levels. The anti-inflammatory action of turmeric is stronger than that of hydrocortisone, and its antioxidant action more powerful than that of vitamin E.

Dose: 2 level teaspoons of powder twice a day during detox (mix into juices and soups).

Other Supplements Used to Boost Liver Detox

Certain substances are protective by helping to reduce the toxic effects of intermediary super-toxins – chemicals produced during the detox process that are more toxic than the original substances. Other supplements used by some practitioners during detox include:

CoEnzyme Q10, available as tablets, protects against toxins, as do sulphur-containing substances found in garlic, onions and cruciferous vegetables.
Dose: Typically 30–90 mg daily

N-acetyl cysteine (NAC) is an amino acid that boosts levels of a powerful antioxidant (glutathione) in the liver and respiratory tract. Interestingly, research is currently under way to investigate observations that NAC can prevent some of the lung damage linked with lung cancer in smokers. Do not take it if you have peptic ulcers.
Dose: 400 mg to 1g daily
Some people might wish to supplement with 250mg glutathione twice daily, or substitute methionine.

Methionine is an essential amino acid that improves the flow of bile from the liver and helps the elimination of fat-soluble toxins. Methionine also prevents glutathione from being depleted.
Dose: 1 g per day.

Kudzu (Pueraria lobata)

Extracts from the roots and flowers of an Indian vine, kudzu, can support liver function by reducing cravings for alcohol. It is also used to treat hangovers.

Dose: 30 mg standardized root 3 times daily.

Supplements to Support Kidney Function

The supplements most commonly used to support kidney function are dandelion and horsetail, which both have a diuretic action.

Dandelion (Taraxacum officinalis)

This plant has long been known for its diuretic properties (see page 40)

Horsetail (Equisetum arvense)

Horsetail is an ancient plant related to trees that grew on Earth 270 million years ago. It has brittle, jointed stems and has been used for centuries to support kidney function, tone the urinary tract and reduce water retention. It reduces sweating, however, this is not always desirable during detox.
Dose: 1g two to three times daily.

Supplements to Support Intestinal Function

Some therapists recommend colonic hydrotherapy during a detox programme in order to help remove toxic waste from the intestines. Unlike an enema, which cleanses only the sigmoid colon (the most distal part of the large intestine), colonic hydrotherapy cleanses the entire large intestine from the downwards. If you prefer, the bowels can be scrubbed clean by eating extra fibre, brushed through with cleansing herbal supplements, flushed by drinking plenty of mineral water and balanced by taking probiotic supplements.

A number of supplements can support intestinal function, including glutamine, fibre supplements, aloe vera, probiotic supplements, chelating agents, garlic, cayenne and ginger.

Aloe vera (Aloe barbadensis)

This succulent plant, native to Africa, has a gel in its fleshy leaves, which contains a unique mix of vitamins, amino acids, enzymes and minerals. These have been valued for their healing properties for over 6,000 years. The gel contains soapy substances (saponins) which help to cleanse the bowel, and pulpy microfibres (lignins) which help to absorb fluid and toxins from the bowel and bulk up the motions. It also

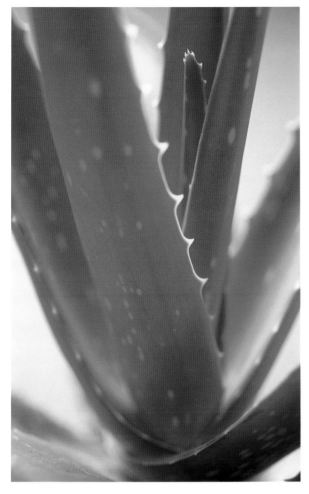

Above: *Aloe vera is a powerful natural laxative*

during detox. Some women notice that it increases their menstrual flow. As it stimulates uterine contractions, it should not be taken during pregnancy or when breast-feeding.

Dose: Start with a small dose (e.g. 1 teaspoon per day) and increase gradually to 1–2 tablespoons per day to find the dose that suits you best. Aloe has a powerful cathartic effect and taking too much will produce a brisk laxative response.

Fibre supplements

Fibre helps digestion by absorbing water in the gut and bulking up the stools. It therefore provides lubrication and a weighty mass that the bowel wall can grip and push downwards in waves of muscular contraction until expelled from the body. Dietary fibre therefore helps to shorten the length of time food stays in the gut and speeds the removal of toxins from the body. Experiments show that for every gram of fibre you eat, your bowel motions increase by around 5 g in weight. This is because dietary fibre provides nutrients for bacterial growth, and much of the increased bowel motion bulk is due to increased bacterial multiplication in the gut. Another benefit of fibre is its ability to absorb toxins from the gut, rather like a sponge, thus decreasing their chance of absorption and increasing their likelihood of excretion.

Fibre-bulking agents are available in a variety of forms, including granules, powders, flakes, husks and natural seeds. These are usually taken once or twice a day with plenty of water. A good fluid intake is essential during detox and when taking fibre supplements because fibre absorbs large quantities of water and can dry the gut out if fluid intake is not increased as well. This can lead to

contains substances that are anti-inflammatory, antioxidant, antiseptic and hasten wound healing.

Aloe vera juice can be made from freshly extracted gel or from powdered aloe (the former is preferable). The fresh gel has to be stabilized within hours of harvesting to prevent oxidation and inactivation. When selecting a product, aim for one made from 100 per cent pure aloe vera. Its strength needs to be at least 40 per cent by volume to be effective, and ideally approaching 95 per cent. You might find it more palatable to choose a product containing a little natural fruit juice to improve the flavour, but some people find that fruit juice makes their symptoms worse.

Aloe vera is an excellent remedy for constipation

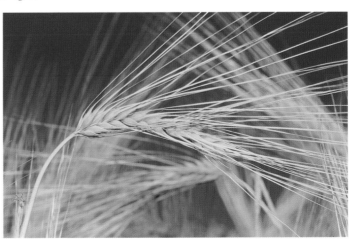

Right: *Fibre helps to gently scrub the bowel clean*

discomfort, bloating and even constipation. Always follow instructions on the pack very carefully.

New research suggests that bowel bacteria adapt to the types of fibre you eat. After a few weeks of a diet rich in, say, bran, the bacteria release more of the enzymes needed to break it down, which means that some of the benefits of taking fibre may be lost. It is therefore worth varying the types of fibre in your diet by eating as wide a range of fibre-rich foods as possible from a variety of sources.

The seeds and husks of Plantago psyllium (guar gum) are considered particularly effective in detox regimes to absorb toxins from the bowel. The presence of a mucilage in the seed husks allows them to swell up to 14 times their original volume when mixed with water. In the intestines, psyllium forms a laxative bulk that gently scrubs the bowel and absorbs toxins and excess fats.

Senna is a stimulant herbal laxative sometimes used to remove toxins rapidly from the bowel. Unless you suffer from constipation, however, it is best avoided. Stimulant laxatives can trigger bowel spasms. Most people following a detox programme will find psyllium more than adequate.
Dose: Follow the recommendations on the packet of whatever supplement you choose.

Fructo-oligosaccarides (FOs)

These naturally occurring forms of carbohydrate, which cannot be digested or absorbed from the human bowel, are classed as probiotic. They act as a fermentable food source for probiotic bacteria and promote their growth in the intestines. By contrast, harmful bacteria such as *E. coli* and *Clostridium*, cannot use FOs as a source of energy. As part of your detox programme, follow an FO-rich diet.

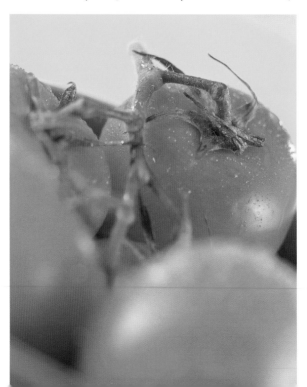

Right: *Tomatoes are an excellent source of FOs*

Dietary sources of FOs

✧ Garlic and onions
✧ Barley and wheat
✧ Bananas
✧ Honey
✧ Tomatoes
✧ Some probiotic supplements

Glutamine

An amino acid made in the body, glutamine nourishes the lining of the intestinal tract, which can use it as a direct source of energy. It can reduce damage to the intestinal tract from dietary and environmental toxins and supports normal gut permeability. Do not take it at night because it is also used as an energy source by the brain, increases alertness and makes it difficult to sleep. Glutamine can also help to reduce cravings for alcohol.
Dose: Around 1 g per day as a stimulant; higher doses of 5–10 g might be recommended during detox.

Humic acids

Chelation is the isolation and removal of heavy metals and other toxic minerals, such as lead and mercury, from the body. Some practitioners – doctors specializing in intravenous chelation therapy – use intravenous chelation to infuse a synthetic amino acid (EDTA) into the bloodstream. This chelates (binds) with heavy metals and other toxic minerals in the circulation to strip them out and excrete them through the kidneys. This regime is not advocated by all, however, as it can also remove nutritionally useful substances. A gentler form of chelation involves taking a colloidal supplement containing certain organic humic acids derived from peat marshes. Humic acids are a rich source of amino acids and can chelate heavy metals in the bowel while at the same time replenishing levels of iron and some trace elements such as selenium, molybdenum and vanadium. Humic acids are excellent detox agents which have been shown to lower levels of toxic lead, mercury, cadmium and caesium.

Substances with a natural chelating effect include aduki beans, lentils and blue-green algae, such as Chlorella, Spirulina and Aphanizomenon flow-aquae (see page 52).

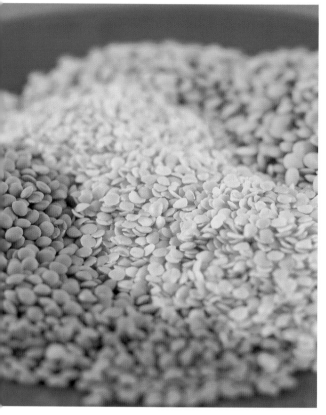

Above: *Lentils have a natural chelating action in the bowel*

Probiotic supplements

Probiotics are widely used for cleansing and replenishing during detox, but few people realize what they are doing when they enjoy that most common probiotic – a live bio yoghurt.

Probiotics is the use of natural bacteria – and substances that promote their growth – to encourage colonization of the bowel by friendly organisms. This creates a healthy intestinal environment that helps to remove toxins, promote healthy digestion and improve local immunity so that the risk of infection with potentially harmful, disease-causing organisms is reduced. In an average toxic person, the number of friendly lactobacilli in the large bowel is typically 15 per cent compared with 85 per cent for unfriendly *E. coli*. Reversing the figures would give the ideal balance. Dietary supplementation with *Lactobacillus acidophilus* and related bio species known to colonize the gut is important during and after a detox programme.

Live bio yoghurt and probiotic supplements contain live cultures of friendly bacteria that help to detoxify the gut by:

✧ producing natural beneficial acids which lower intestinal pH and discourage reproduction of less acid-tolerant, harmful bacteria and yeast infections

✧ secreting natural antibiotics that compete with harmful bacteria for available nutrients

✧ competing with other bacteria to attach to intestinal cell walls – literally crowding them out so that they pass through the intestines and are eliminated before they can gain a foothold

✧ stimulating production of interferon, a natural anti-viral agent which helps to protect against viral intestinal infections

✧ overcoming constipation and improving elimination

✧ inhibiting the growth of *Helicobacter pylori*, a bacterium linked with gastritis, gastric ulcers and stomach cancer

✧ reducing the formation of cancer-causing substances in the gut by inhibiting the enzymes necessary to produce them

✧ reducing the absorption of ammonia from the intestines

✧ boosting the function of immune cells, such as phagocytes, lymphocytes and natural killer cells

✧ promoting the production of protective antibodies by acting as an antigen donor

✧ inhibiting bacterial enzymes used to produce cancer-causing substances in the large bowel

✧ countering the development of allergies

✧ reducing symptoms of lactose intolerance in susceptible individuals

Probiotic bacteria have been shown to have a protective effect against a number of toxic bacteria, including *Salmonella typhi*, *E. coli* and *Candida albicans*.

Unfortunately, probiotic bacteria are fragile and bio yoghurt that has been sitting in the supermarket or in your fridge for a week or more will contain less live bacteria than freshly made cultures. There should be at least one million live bifidobacterium and/or one million live acidophilus bacteria per gram of yoghurt for maximum detox potential. Levels of live probiotic bacteria in bio yoghurts vary widely, however, from a few hundred thousand to more than 300 million live bacteria per gram. For this reason, it is best to take a probiotic supplement as part of your detox programme.

When choosing a supplement, select one that supplies at least 10 million–2 billion colony-forming units (CFU) of acidophilus per dose. To maintain a high population of probiotic bacteria in your gut, you should ideally take a probiotic supplement for at least a month and repeat this regularly throughout the year whenever you feel your intestinal function has started to deteriorate.

Sources of probiotic bacteria

✧ Live bio yoghurt; yoghurts labelled merely "live" might contain only bacteria such as *Streptococcus thermophilus*, which are not found naturally in the human body and are usually killed during digestion.
✧ Fermented milk drinks containing lactobacilli
✧ Supplements that guarantee a specified potency of bacteria in capsule, powder, liquid or tablet form; these should ideally be kept refrigerated
✧ Home-made yoghurt produced with freeze-dried acidophilus

Who needs probiotic bacteria?

If any of the following are part of your life, the chances are that you are deficient in probiotic bacteria and would benefit from taking a supplement.

- a nutrient-poor diet
- a recent course of antibiotics
- intestinal problems, such as irritable bowel syndrome, inflammatory bowel disease, chronic diarrhoea, diverticulitis
- recurrent candida or other bowel infections
- serious illness
- reduced immunity

Mercury

Mercury is a highly toxic metal found in pesticides and fungicides, fish (especially tuna) from polluted waters, industrial waste and dental amalgams.

It is important to avoid having mercury amalgam tooth fillings removed or inserted during detox. Later, you might wish to consult a dentist who specializes in the removal of mercury fillings. Teeth are usually restored in quadrants – one quarter of the mouth at a time – and supplements that bind to mercury and help to eliminate it from the body should be taken. It is estimated that for every year mercury amalgams have been in your mouth, it will take a month for your body to detox itself and for all mercury to be removed from the tissues.

Garlic (Allium sativum)

See page 40.

Cayenne (Capsicum frutescens)

Cayenne, or chilli pepper, is a perennial shrub native to Mexico, but is now found throughout the tropics, especially in Africa and India. Its scarlet fruits filled with white seed are familiar in kitchens worldwide. The ingredient that imparts spiciness to the pods is capsaicin. The seeds also contain steroidal saponins known as capsicidins.

Cayenne stimulates the circulation and promotes sweating. It also aids the digestion by promoting the elimination of toxins from the gut by encouraging the production of intestinal mucus.

Dose: 500–1,000 mg per day in capsule or tablet form; 1–2 ml as a tincture.

Ginger (Zingiber officinale)

This perennial, tropical plant forms knobbly, thickened structures known as tuberous rhizomes, which put out attractive, lance-shaped green and purple leaves. Ginger is one of the oldest medicinal spices known. It has analgesic, antihistamine, anti-inflammatory and anti-nausea actions, plus a warming effect that promotes sweating, all of which make it useful for detox. Its antiseptic action can support healthy bowel bacteria, such as lactobacilli, while discouraging undesirable bowel infections.

Ginger was recently found to act like garlic in reducing blood-clotting, boosting the circulation and lowering blood pressure. It can be used to quell nausea during toxic detox and to relieve headaches, indigestion, bloating and diarrhoea.

Dose: 7.5g fresh ginger (sliced and bruised or grated) steeped in a mug of boiling water for five minutes. Add organic honey and lemon to taste.

250 mg powdered ginger root capsules standardized for 0.4 per cent volatile oils, 2–4 times per day.

Cleansing homeopathic supplements

Homoeopathy is one of the most popular forms of complementary medicine. It is based on two major

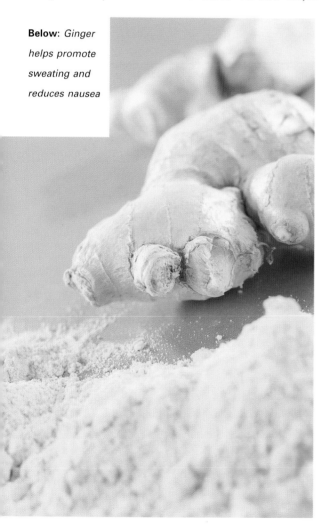

Below: *Ginger helps promote sweating and reduces nausea*

principles. The first, that "like cures like", means that substances that cause particular symptoms will also cure them. The second, that "less cures more", means that the tinier the dose, the greater its effect. By diluting substances many hundreds, thousands or even millions of times, their healing properties are enhanced while any undesirable side effects are lost.

Homoeopathic remedies are prepared from mother tinctures, which are mixed on a decimal or centesimal scale: one part tincture to nine parts alcohol becomes the 1x potency, while one part tincture to 99 parts alcohol becomes the 1c potency. The process continues, taking one part of each dilution and mixing it with either nine or 99 parts alcohol until the required potency is reached. To illustrate just how dilute these substances are, a dilution of 12c is comparable to a pinch of salt dissolved in the same volume of water as the Atlantic Ocean.

How to take homoeopathic remedies

Homoeopathic remedies, usually in pill or tablet form, should be taken no less than 10 minutes before or after eating or drinking. Transfer them to the mouth without handling them by tipping them into the lid of the container or on to a teaspoon. Allow the pills to dissolve under the tongue – don't swallow them whole.

A form of homoeopathy known as drainage is helpful when following a detox regime. This aims to stimulate one or more of the natural excretory organs of the body to assist in the cleansing of toxins. It provides support for the liver, kidneys, lungs, skin, lymph vessels and mucous membranes.

A remedy known as the "drainer complex" can be taken for one or two weeks during detox. It contains six homoeopathic elements to assist elimination: Bryonia, Nux vomica, Berberis, Chelidonium, Solidago and Taraxacum.

A number of other homoeopathic remedies can also be used to assist drainage. These should be individually tailored to your needs, so it is important to consult a qualified homoeopathic practitioner.

FUNCTION	HOMOEOPATHIC DRAINERS
To stimulate the adrenal glands	Adrenalin
To stimulate the lymphatics	Phytolacca
To stimulate mucous membranes	Allium cepa, Euphrasia, Hydrastis, Kalium iodatum, Ledum, Sabadilla
To assist liver function	Bryonia, Carduus marianus, Chelidonium, Cinchona, Conium, Nux vomica, Secale, Solidago, Taraxacum
To assist kidney function	Berberis, Formica rufa, Sarsaparilla, Solidago,
To assist skin function	Calendula, Fumaria, Saponaria, Petroleum, Viola tricolor
To assist lung function	Sticta
To assist intestinal function	Condurango, Ornithogallium, Ruta graveolens

Detoxing with acupuncture

Acupuncture is an ancient therapy based on the belief that life energy (*ch'i* or *qi*, pronounced "chee") flows through your body along different channels called meridians. This flow of energy depends on the balance of two opposing forces – yin and yang – a balance which is easily disrupted through factors such as stress, emotional upset, poor diet and spiritual neglect. When the energy flow becomes blocked, symptoms of illness are triggered.

There are twelve main meridians, six of which have a yang polarity and are related to hollow organs, such as the womb, and six of which are yin, relating mainly to solid organs, such as the liver. Eight further meridians control the other twelve. Along each meridian a number of acupoints have been identified where ch'i energy is concentrated and can enter or leave the body. Three hundred and sixty-five classic acupoints were traditionally sited on the meridians, but many more have now been discovered, and around two thousand acupoints are illustrated on modern charts.

Acupuncture using five acupoints in the ear (auricular therapy) can be used during detox to help overcome cravings for such things as sweets, fatty foods, nicotine, caffeine, alcohol or drugs.

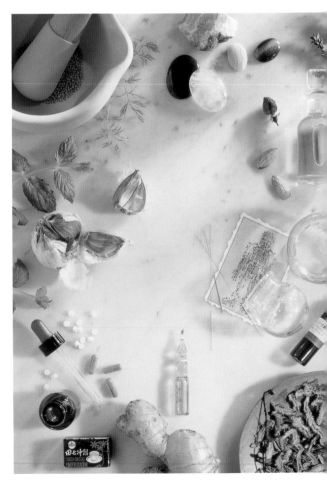

Above: *A variety of herbal and homeopathic preparations can aid detox*

Giving up smoking

Nicotine, the addictive constituent of tobacco, is a poison that can produce withdrawal symptoms of tension, aggression, depression, insomnia and cravings. You therefore need to take things slowly and perhaps work at cutting down and stopping smoking before starting a full detox plan.

Tips to help you stop smoking

❖ Find support – giving up smoking is easier with a friend or partner.

❖ Cut out a number of cigarettes per day, starting with those you will miss the least.

❖ Continue reducing your intake until you stop gradually, or until you feel ready to cut out the remaining cigarettes altogether.

❖ Name the day to quit and get into the right frame of mind.

❖ Remove temptation by throwing away all tobacco supplies, smoking papers, matches, lighters and ashtrays.

❖ Concentrate on getting through each day – try not to think long term, which can be daunting.

❖ When you want to smoke, think positive by saying to yourself, "While I would like a cigarette, I don't need one because I no longer smoke," then remind yourself of all the reasons you have decided to quit.

❖ Keep a detox smoking chart and tick off every day you keep within your target level of consumption or have lasted without a cigarette.

❖ Plan a reward for every week of success.

❖ Relax with massage, yoga or meditation.

❖ Keep your hands busy with model-making, drawing, painting, embroidery or origami.

❖ Increase the amount of regular exercise you take, as this can help to curb withdrawal symptoms.

❖ Identify situations where you would usually smoke and either avoid them or plan ahead to overcome them. For example, practise saying, "No, thanks, I've given up," or "No, thanks, I'm cutting down".

❖ Ask friends and relatives not to smoke around you.

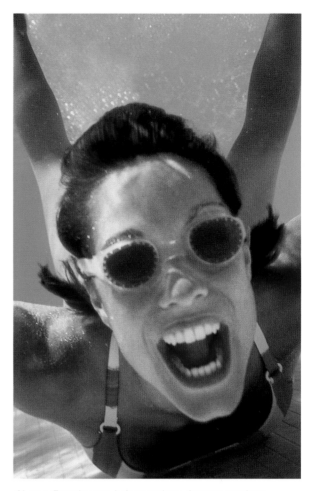

Above: *Exercise can help to reduce cigarette cravings*

Tips to help you overcome cravings

❖ Suck on an artificial cigarette or herbal stick available from chemist shops.

❖ Suck on celery or carrot sticks.

❖ Eat an apple.

❖ Clean your teeth with strongly flavoured toothpaste.

❖ Go out for a brisk walk, swim, cycle-ride or jog.

❖ Take a supplement containing oat straw (*Avena sativa*) which can reduce cravings.

❖ Take a flower essence, such as Rescue Remedy, Emergency Essence or Agrimony (*Agrimonia eupatoria*). For those who seek solace in drugs or alcohol, crab apple (*Malus pumila*) helps to detoxify and cleanse.

❖ Use essential oil products, such as Logado or Nicobrevin, to reduce cravings.

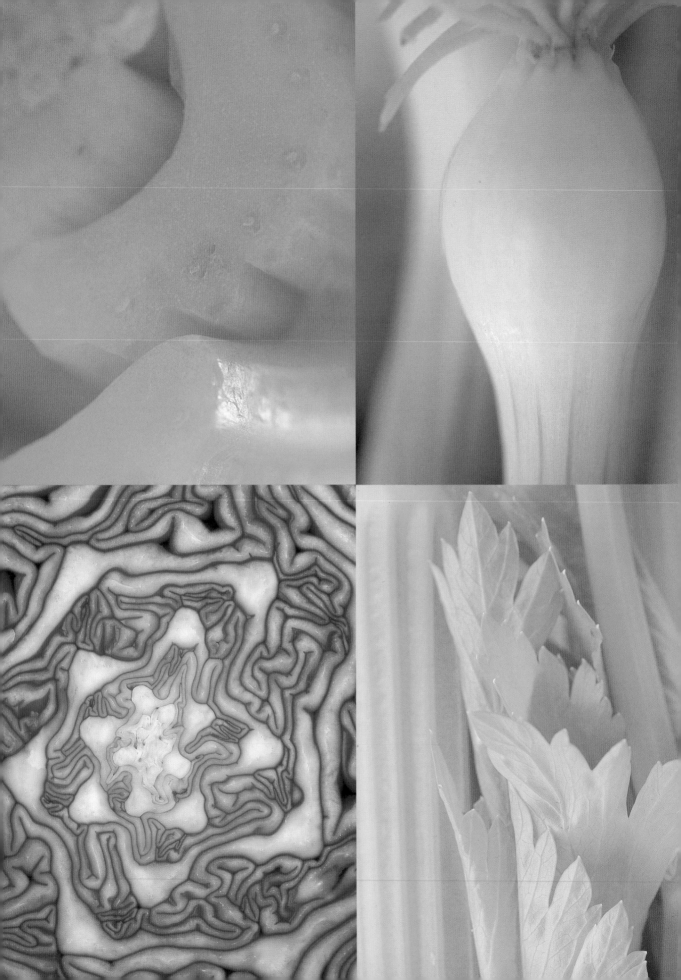

Once your cleansing programme is under way, you can start providing balance by adding in nutritional supplements. These provide important vitamins, minerals and essential fatty acids that can help your body achieve optimal nutritional balance.

CHAPTER FOUR

Balance

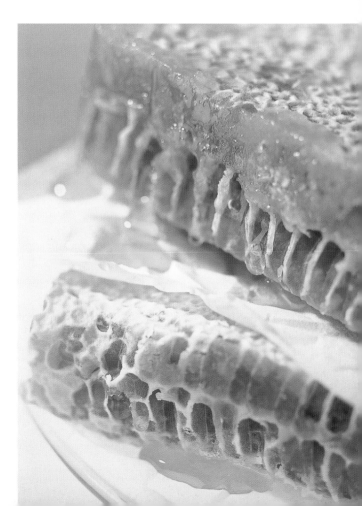

The classic rationale of detox is that nutrient supplements (apart from antioxidants and acidophilus sources) are not started immediately – just as you would not add new oil when servicing a car until the old, dirty oil (the toxins) have first been drained away. You therefore cleanse first, then fortify with vitamin and mineral supplements plus essential fatty acids, such as evening primrose or omega-3 fish oils.

To help achieve balance, one of a number of adaptogens (e.g. a herb, like one of the ginsengs) will help the body adapt to, or cope with times of stress and illness and is often recommended to help your body cope with and adapt to the detox process.

In the long term, balance also comes from following a healthier diet and lifestyle to reduce the future build up of toxins. A healthy, balanced diet should ideally contain wholegrains, vegetables, pulses, white meat and fish with very little sugar, salt, caffeine or alcohol. The desire for sweet things can be satisfied by eating more fresh and dried fruits, or organic honey.

Several complementary therapies are also available to help you to maintain balance once the cleansing process is over.

Nutritional Supplements

Once the detox process is complete, it's time to rebuild the nutritional foundations of health and well-being. While diet should always come first, a significant number of people do not obtain all the vitamins, minerals and essential fatty acids they need from their food. In the case of some vital nutrients, such as selenium, our soils are so depleted that even when eating a healthy organic diet, it is almost impossible to obtain the quantities required to help protect against cancer from food alone. It is therefore sensible to consider taking a multivitamin and mineral supplement, and evening primrose oil for essential fatty acids. You should also consider taking an additional antioxidant supplement (see page 37) and a probiotic supplement, and think about taking chlorophyll-containing algae. If you are lacking in energy, you might also wish to consider coenzyme-Q10. All these supplements are described more fully in the pages following.

Algae

Spirulina, chlorella and blue-green algae such as aphanizomenon flow-aquae evolved over 3.5 billion years ago as the first successful life form on Earth. They had the planet to themselves for 1,000 million years, and chlorella became the first form of life to develop a true cell nucleus, which spirulina and blue-green algae lack. It represents a wholefood source of over 100 synergistic and easily assimilated nutrients, including antioxidants, vitamins, minerals, enzymes, essential fatty acids, essential and non-essential amino acids, iron, chlorophyll, protein and other protective substances. As the basis for the development of life on Earth, algae are one of the most easily assimilable foods for the human body. Their proteins, for example, are in the form of glyco-proteins, which the body prefers to those found as lipoproteins in most foods because it does not have to expend energy converting them into a useable form.

Research by the US space agency NASA suggests that blue-green algae are the perfect food for astronauts as they are the most nutrient-dense food on the planet, providing more vitamins, minerals and protein per acre than any other food source. But even Earthlings can benefit: you take as much as you like during the balancing part of the detox process.

Algae also have a useful chelating action in the body (see page 44). The blue phytochemical found in spirulina, for example, has a powerful detoxifying action that helps to reduce kidney damage due to heavy metals, such as mercury. *Dose*: Varies from product to product, but typically 3 g per day. Large amounts can be consumed as a food without apparent harm. Some products have been contaminated with toxic algae, so ensure you take a recognized, mainstream brand – preferably one grown in unpolluted waters and certified organic.

Algae are good for you!
Although algae might look like simple forms of life, they have a wealth of nutrients. Aphanizomenon flos-aquae, for example, contains:

68% protein

23% carbohydrate

3% fats

11 vitamins, including betacarotene, vitamin B12, folic acid

27 elements, including calcium, iron, zinc

11 pigments, including carotenoids

All eight essential amino acids in optimum proportions

10 other non-essential amino acids

A variety of co-factors and enzymes

Nucleic acids

Essential fatty acids

As well as supplying nutrients, algae have a useful detoxifying action. When toxins such as mercury, copper, lead and cadmium are added to yeast cultures, for example, the cells start to die. If chlorella is added, however, the yeast cells survive because algae have an amazing ability to absorb and neutralize toxins – they can even bind uranium.

Chlorophyll in blue-green algae closely resembles the structure of haemoglobin in our own blood, but where haemoglobin has an iron atom, chlorophyll has magnesium.

Evening Primrose Oil

The seeds of the evening primrose (*Oenothera biennis*) are a rich source of an essential fatty acid (EFA) called gamma linolenic acid (GLA), which acts as a building block for healthy skin and hormone balance. It also has an anti-inflammatory action. EFAs cannot be synthesized in the body, and must therefore come from the diet. They are so important for metabolic balance that at one time they were collectively known as vitamin F. Unfortunately, it is estimated that eight out of ten people are deficient in EFAs because they do not eat enough nuts, seeds and oily fish.

There are two main essential fatty acids. Linolenic acid, of which gamma-linolenic acid is one type, is found in evening primrose oil, starflower (borage) seed oil and blackcurrant seed oil; linoleic acid is found in sunflower seeds, almonds, corn, sesame seeds, safflower oil and extra virgin olive oil. Both linolenic and linoleic acids are found in rich quantities in walnuts, pumpkin seeds, soybeans, linseed oil, rapeseed oil and flax oil.

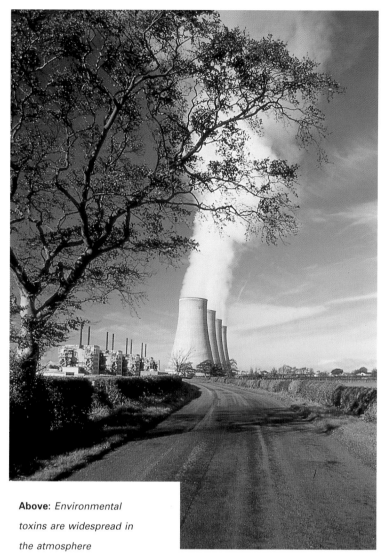

Above: *Environmental toxins are widespread in the atmosphere*

Once in the body, EFAs are fed into a series of metabolic reactions (the EFA pathway) that convert them into hormone-like substances called prostaglandins. Prostaglandins are involved in a variety of balancing metabolic reactions. Some gamma-linolenic acid can be synthesized from dietary linoleic acid, but this reaction needs an enzyme (delta-6-desaturase) that is easily blocked by a number of factors associated with an unhealthy diet and lifestyle. These include excessive intakes of saturated (animal) fat, trans-fatty acids (as found in hydrogenated margarines), sugar and alcohol, a lack of vitamins and minerals, especially vitamin B6, zinc and magnesium, crash dieting, smoking cigarettes and exposure to pollution.

When you do not get enough essential fatty acids from your diet, the metabolism can make do with the next best fatty acids available, such as those derived from saturated fats, but as a result, prostaglandin imbalances are common. Prostaglandins made from other sorts of fat cannot be converted into prostaglandins made from EFAs. This increases the risk of imbalances, especially in sex hormones, and is linked with dry, itchy skin, chronic inflammatory diseases, such as rheumatoid arthritis, psoriasis and eczema, and gynaecological problems, such as cyclical breast pain. Taking an evening primrose oil supplement overcomes any enzyme blocks by feeding into the middle of the EFA pathway.

Fatigue and exhaustion are also common effects of toxicity, and in one trial, EFA supplements produced significant benefits within three months in 90 per cent of people suffering from chronic fatigue.

Dose: 1,000mg per day for general health. Up to 3g per day may be taken to treat hormone imbalances, such as those associated with cyclical breast pain, premenstrual syndrome or menopausal symptoms. It can take up to three months to notice a beneficial effect.

The action of GLA is boosted by vitamin E. Certain vitamins and minerals are also needed during the metabolism of essential fatty acids. These are vitamin C, vitamin B6, vitamin B3 (niacin), zinc and magnesium. If you are taking evening primrose oil, you should therefore ensure that your intake of these is adequate.

The only people who should not take evening primrose oil are those who are allergic to it, and those with a particular nervous disorder known as temporal lobe epilepsy.

Multivitamins and minerals

Select a vitamin and mineral supplement that provides around 100 per cent of the recommended daily amount (RDA) of as many vitamins and minerals as possible. You will also be taking an additional antioxidant supplement.

Although needed in only minute amounts, vitamins and minerals are nutrients which are essential for health and well-being. They are involved in speeding up reactions that digest food, unharness oxygen, produce energy, allow cells to grow, fight infection and keep the metabolism ticking over smoothly. Minerals also play a structural role in bones and teeth. Some vitamins and minerals act as antioxidants (see page 37) and protect the body from some of the harmful effects of toxins.

The following table shows the recommended daily amount (RDA) for a variety of vitamins and minerals. Higher intakes of some (e.g. vitamins C and E and minerals calcium and selenium) are increasingly recommended by some nutritionists.

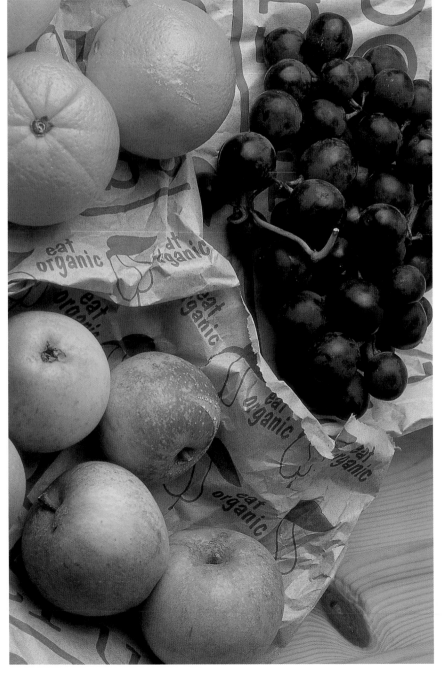

Left: *Organic produce is less likely to contain toxins than those farmed non-organically*

VITAMIN	RDA	FUNCTION	GOOD SOURCES
A	800 mcg	Regulates the way genes are read to make proteins. Controls normal growth and development. Maintains healthy skin and mucous membranes. Needed for night vision.	Animal and fish liver, eggs, oily fish, milk, cheese, butter margarine. Betacarotene (two vitamin A molecules joined together) is found in dark green leafy vegetables and yellow-orange fruits.
B1	1.4 mg	B group vitamins are needed for energy production in cells, healthy nerve function, cell division and immunity.	Brewer's yeast, yeast extract, brown rice, wheatgerm and wheat bran, nuts, wholegrain cereals, meat, seafood, liver, dairy products, green, leafy vegetables.
B2	1.6 mg		
B3	18 mg		
B5	6 mg		
B6	2 mg		
B12	1 mcg		
Biotin	0.15 mg	Produced by friendly bowel bacteria. Needed for healthy hair, skin and sweat glands. Involved in metabolism and the formation of energy storage molecules.	Liver, kidney, yeast extract, nuts, wholegrain cereals.
Folate	200 mcg	Essential for normal cell division and healthy nerve function. Protects against some developmental abnormalities, such as spina bifida, during early pregnancy; lowers levels of homocysteine – an amino acid linked with hardening and furring up of the arteries.	Green, leafy vegetables, yeast extract, wholegrains, nuts, liver, dairy products, citrus fruits, eggs.
C	60 mg	Involved in making collagen, an important structural protein. Needed for healthy tissues, growth, repair and reproduction.	Citrus fruits, blackcurrants, kiwi fruit, mangoes, green peppers, green, leafy vegetables, parsley and other green herbs.
D	5 mcg	Needed for absorption of calcium and phosphate from the diet. Essential for healthy bones and teeth.	Oily fish (e.g. sardines, herring, mackerel, salmon, tuna), fish liver oils, margarine, liver, eggs, fortified milk.
E	10 mg	A powerful antioxidant that protects body fats (e.g. cell membranes, nerve sheaths and cholesterol molecules) from damage. Strengthens muscle fibres, boosts immunity and improves skin suppleness and healing.	Wheatgerm oil, avocados, nuts, seeds, margarine, eggs, butter, wholegrains, oily fish.

MINERAL	RDA	FUNCTION	GOOD SOURCES
Calcium	800 mg	Major component of bones and teeth. Essential for nerve conduction, muscle contraction and energy production. Needed for blood-clotting, some enzyme actions and immune functions.	Milk and dairy products, green, leafy vegetables, salmon, nuts and seeds, pulses, eggs.
Iodine	150 mcg	Produces two thyroid hormones, which control the metabolic rate.	Fish (e.g. haddock, salmon, tuna), seafood (e.g. prawns, mussels, lobster, oysters), seaweed, iodized salt, milk.
Iron	14 mg	Needed for the production of haemoglobin, the red pigment that transports oxygen around the body. Also found in myoglobin, which binds oxygen in muscle cells. Needed to produce energy and for fighting infections.	Red meat, fish (especially sardines), brewer's yeast, offal, wheatgerm, wholemeal bread, egg yolk, green vegetables, parsley and other green herbs, prunes and other dried fruit.
Magnesium	300 mg	Maintains the electrical stability of cells and regulates heartbeat. Needed for most metabolic reactions – few enzymes can work without it.	Soya, nuts, brewer's yeast, wholegrains, brown rice, seafood, meat, eggs, dairy products, bananas, dark green, leafy vegetables, herbs, chocolate.
Phosphorus	800 mg	A major component of bones and teeth. Essential for the production of energy-rich storage compounds.	Milk and dairy products, nuts, wholegrain cereals, poultry, eggs, meat, fish, legumes.
Zinc	15 mg	Essential for the proper function of over 100 enzymes. Vital for growth, sexual maturity, wound-healing and immunity.	Red meat, seafood (especially oysters), offal, brewer's yeast, wholegrains, pulses, eggs, cheese.

Omega-3 fish oils

Derived from the flesh rather than the liver of oily fish, omega-3 fish oils contain essential fatty acids (eicosapentaenoic acid) which have a beneficial effect on liver function and blood fats to reduce the risk of hardening and furring up of the arteries, heart attack, high blood pressure and stroke.

Some research suggests fish oils increase blood sugar levels in diabetics. However, omega-3 fish oils protect against the increased risk of coronary heart disease that occurs in diabetes. If diabetic, monitor sugar levels carefully while taking fish oil supplements.

Dose: Usually 1–4 g per day. Added vitamin E stops the content of the capsules becoming rancid.

Getting your diet right

A healthy, balancing diet should provide all the energy, protein, essential fatty acids, vitamins, minerals and co-factors your body needs without providing any to excess. Unfortunately, many foods contain pesticides, fertilizers, growth enhancers and other agricultural chemicals that are strongly suspected of having toxic effects in the body. As part of your long-term detox plan, it is vitally important to eat as organically as possible (see page 33).

Foods rich in antioxidants (such as vegetables, nuts and seeds), beans and wholegrains,

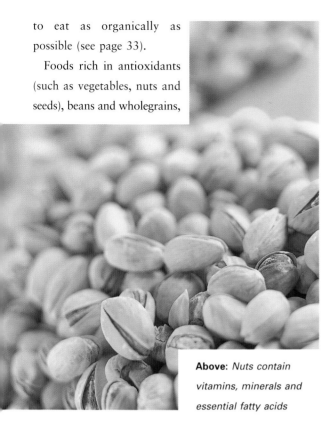

Above: *Nuts contain vitamins, minerals and essential fatty acids*

carotenoids (green, yellow and orange fruits and vegetables), bioflavonoids (found together with vitamin C in most fruit and vegetables), and cruciferous vegetables (cabbage, Brussels sprouts, cauliflower and broccoli), all help to improve your detoxification systems.

Apart from improving what you eat, it is also important to change how you eat:

✧ Eat fruit and vegetables raw, or just lightly steamed, as appropriate.

✧ Eat little and often rather than having two or three big meals per day.

✧ Chew your food well, as this releases enzymes which help in digestion.

✧ Avoid processed foods, additives, sugar, salt, caffeine and alcohol as much as possible.

Carbohydrate

Dietary carbohydrates are the body's main source of energy and should ideally provide at least half your daily energy intake. Complex, unrefined carbohydrates, such as wholegrain cereals, brown rice, wholemeal bread, wholewheat pasta and jacket potatoes, are preferable because they contain additional valuable nutrients, such as vitamins, trace elements and dietary fibre.

Some forms of carbohydrate are known to cause large swings in circulating blood glucose levels which can trigger unwanted toxic effects to metabolism and health. The extent to which they do this is known as their glycaemic index (GI). For general health – and especially when following a detox plan – try to select foods with a low to moderate GI. Foods with a high GI should be combined with those providing a lower GI value to reduce blood sugar level fluctuations. Root vegetables, for example, combine well with kidney beans.

GLYCAEMIC INDEX OF WHOLEFOODS

(Glucose = 100)

Food	GI
Baked potatoes	98
Parsnips	97
Carrots	92
Honey	87
Brown rice	82
Wholemeal bread	72
Raisins	64
Bananas	62
Sweetcorn	59
Sweet potatoes	50
Oats	49
Grapes	44
Wholemeal pasta	42
Organic baked beans	40
Oranges	40
Apples	39
Butter beans	36
Chick peas	36
Milk	32
Haricot beans	31
Apricots	30
Kidney beans	29
Lentils	29
Peaches	29
Grapefruit	26
Barley	22
Soy beans	15

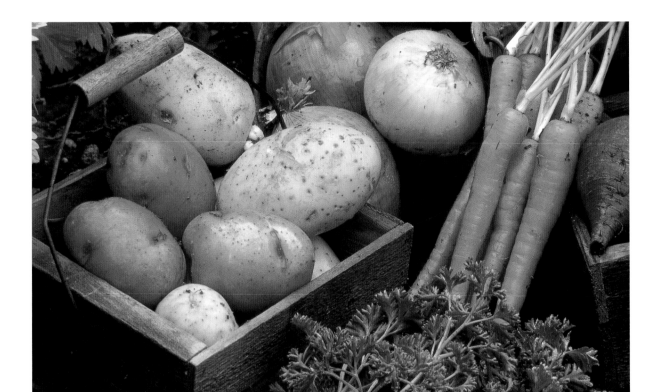

Above: *Aim to eat at least five, preferably ten, pieces of fruit and vegetables each day*

To maximize energy levels, minimize fat storage and stabilize blood glucose levels it helps to eat five or six small meals or snacks a day at regularly spaced intervals.

Dietary fats

A certain amount of fat is important for healthy cell membranes, nerve function and hormone balance. A diet that provides too much fat, and not enough starchy foods or fruit and vegetables is harmful to health. Balance is therefore vitally important. Fats are the richest dietary source of energy but should ideally provide no more than 30 per cent of your daily energy intake. Essential fatty acids, which are vital for health, cannot be made in the body, so they must come from dietary sources, such as nuts, seeds, green, leafy vegetables, oily fish and wholegrain cereals, or by taking supplements such as evening primrose oil or omega-3 fish oils (see pages 53 and 56).

A balancing diet should ideally contain fish – especially oily fish, such as mackerel, sardines and salmon. These are rich in eicosapentanoic acid (EPA), a substance that thins the blood, lowers cholesterol levels, reduces high blood pressure and protects against coronary heart disease. EPA

also controls inflammation and can reduce the toxic effects of inflammatory conditions, such as rheumatoid arthritis, ulcerative colitis, psoriasis and possibly asthma. Fish oils have also been found to halt the growth of certain cancer cells, reduce the risk of intestinal polyps and reverse weight loss in cancer patients. The British Nutritional Foundation suggests that we eat at least 300 g (11 oz) of oily fish per week (2–3 servings), which, at current estimates, means increasing our average intake by a factor of 10. It is important, however, to buy fish farmed from seas declared organic by the Soil Association to avoid increasing your intake of toxins that might be found in fish caught in polluted waters.

Olive oil is a rich source of oleic acid, a mono-unsaturated fat that keeps blood cholesterol levels healthy and reduces the risk of coronary heart disease. It might also help to protect against gallstones.

Protein

Proteins are made up of building blocks or amino acids, of which 20 are important for human health. Of these, 10 nutritionally essential amino acids cannot be synthesized in the body in adequate amounts and must be derived from food.

Essential Amino Acids

- Arginine
- Histidine
- Isoleucine
- Leucine
- Lysine
- Methionine
- Phenylalanine
- Threonine
- Tryptophan
- Valine
- Tyrosine (synthesized from phenylalanine)
- Cysteine (synthesized from methionine)

Non-essential Amino Acids

- Alanine
- Asparagine
- Aspartic acid
- Glutamine
- Glutamic acid
- Glycine
- Proline
- Serine

Dietary protein can be divided into two groups. First-class proteins provide significant amounts of the essential amino acids from meat, fish, eggs and dairy products. Second-class proteins contain some, but not all, essential amino acids from foods such as vegetables, rice, beans and nuts.

During some detox programmes, intakes of first-class proteins derived from animal sources (e.g. red meat) are often reduced. As simple detox diets recommend eating wholegrain rice and a wide variety of vegetables and pulses, intakes of second-class proteins that mix and match the essential amino acids are usually adequate. Those following long-term detox eating plans are usually able to obtain a balanced protein intake by eating five parts rice to one part beans.

Fruit and Vegetables

The importance of fruit, vegetables, nuts, seeds and pulses in the diet can hardly be overstated. They are rich sources of vitamins, minerals, fibre and at least 20 non-nutrient substances, known as phytochemicals, which help to protect health and immunity. Some of these substances are powerful antioxidants, while others have beneficial hormone-like actions or anti-inflammatory effects in the body.

Many studies suggest that those who eat the most raw and fresh fruit (including tomatoes) are least likely to develop coronary heart disease and cancer. The exact reason is unknown, but is probably due to a variety of beneficial substances found in fruit. These include flavonoids, soluble fibre, micronutrients, phytochemicals and phytoestrogens.

Flavonoids are natural antioxidants that help to maintain health and protect against disease. They protect cell membranes from damage and also help to prevent hardening and furring up of the arteries. Almost every fruit and vegetable contains flavonoids, of which over 20,000 are known to exist. One study found that men who ate the most flavonoids had less than half the number of fatal heart attacks compared with those who ate the least. The chief sources of flavonoids in the study were apples, onions and tea.

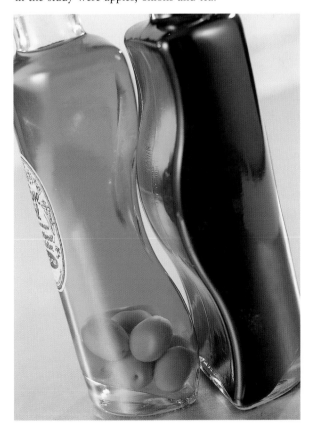

Above: *Olive oil has beneficial effects on the circulation*

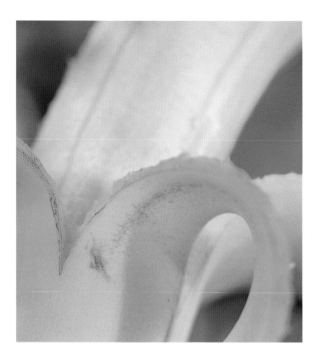

Left: *Bananas are a source of phytoestrogens*

in their own right. As a result, phytoestrogens are helpful for a variety of female problems, including menopausal symptoms, premenstrual syndrome, endometriosis and fibroids. They also seem to protect against some hormone-dependent tumours, such as breast cancer. Fresh fruits that are known to contain phytoestrogens include apples, avocados, bananas, mangoes, papaya, dates, figs, prunes and raisins.

Eating an apple a day might keep the doctor away, after all.

TOP FOODS FOR A BALANCING DIET

Apricots Like all yellow, orange and green fruit and vegetables, apricots are a rich source of antioxidant carotenoids, as well as vitamin C, iron, potassium and fibre.

Broccoli Dark green vegetables, such as broccoli, spinach and spring greens, are rich in vitamin C, folic acid and calcium. Broccoli also contains phytochemicals, which have a powerful anti-cancer effect, especially against tumours of the digestive tract, lungs, breast and prostate gland.

Cherries These contain a phytochemical called ellagic acid, which protects against cancer by blocking an enzyme needed for the growth of cancer cells. Cherries have a mild laxative action and also help to prevent gout. A good source of vitamin C and potassium.

Chillies Eating chillies stimulates production of mucus in the stomach, which might protect against peptic ulcers

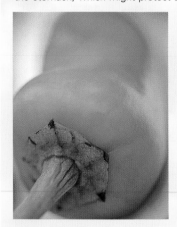

and help to expel toxins. Chillies also contain antioxidants, which help to protect against coronary heart disease, cancer and premature ageing. Phytochemicals in chilli peppers thin the blood to reduce

Soluble fibre helps to keep the bowels working normally. A number of studies have found that those eating more fruit are less likely to suffer from cancer of the colon.

Micronutrients contain all the important vitamins, minerals and trace elements you need. They are good sources of vitamins C and E, betacarotene and mineral selenium. Fruit also contains potassium, which helps to flush excess sodium through the kidneys and might help to reduce high blood pressure. Yellow, orange and red fruits are rich sources of betacarotene, a natural pigment related to vitamin A, which seems to protect against cancer. Ideally, we need to obtain 6 mg of betacarotene per day (from food rather than supplements), but most of us obtain only about 2 mg daily.

Phytochemicals are protective plant chemicals that seem to help protect against cancer by blocking an enzyme needed for the growth of cancer cells. Fruit and vegetables particularly rich in phytochemicals include apricots, cherries, grapes, onions, tomatoes, garlic and parsley.

Phytoestrogens are plant hormones that have a weak, oestrogen-like effect in the body. They reduce the effects of excess oestrogen by knocking stronger oestrogens off their receptors, but can also boost low levels of oestrogen

the risk of blood clots, high blood pressure and raised cholesterol levels. They are a good source of betacarotene and vitamin C.

Citrus fruits An excellent source of vitamin C (vital for healthy bones and skin) and bioflavonoids (powerful antioxidants that help to protect against cancer, heart disease and inflammation). Citrus fruits also contain pectin, a soluble fibre that helps to lower high cholesterol levels. Lemons are a rich source of limonene, a phytochemical that protects against cancer. Using lime juice as a flavouring reduces the need for salt.

Cranberry juice Research suggests that drinking 300 ml (½ pint) cranberry juice per day almost halves the risk of cystitis. Cranberries contain phytochemicals (known as anti-adhesins) that stop bacteria and toxins sticking to the wall of the urinary tract, so they are flushed out more easily. Also a good source of vitamin C.

Garlic The phytochemicals contained in garlic protect against high cholesterol levels and high blood pressure, improve the circulation and reduce the risk of coronary heart disease and stroke. Studies in China suggest that those who regularly eat up to 20 g (¾ oz) fresh garlic per day have the lowest rate of stomach cancer. Garlic is a natural decongestant and its antiviral and antibacterial actions help keep coughs and colds at bay.

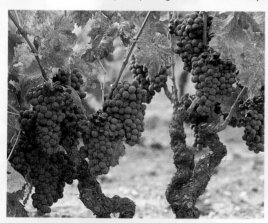

Grapes Like cherries, grapes contain ellagic acid, which has powerful anti-cancer properties. Red and black grapes also contain antioxidant pigments, which are more powerful than vitamins C or E. Resveratrol, for example, helps to prevent hardening and furring up of the arteries. Grapes are a good source of potassium and of trace minerals, such as boron, magnesium and copper.

Papaya Also known as paw-paw, papaya is an excellent source of betacarotene, vitamin C and fibre. It contains an enzyme, papain, which breaks down protein and boosts digestion. Because the flesh is soft and easily digested, it is an excellent food for convalescence. The seeds taste like peppercorns and can be dried and ground to make a healthy, spicy seasoning.

Parsley A good source of vitamin C, iron and folic acid. Parsley is used in medical herbalism as a mild diuretic, to stimulate menstruation, to boost digestion and ease colic and wind.

Red peppers An excellent source of vitamin C, betacarotene and bioflavonoids. Weight for weight, red peppers contain three times as much vitamin C as citrus fruits (green peppers – the unripened form of red peppers – have over twice as much).

Rhubarb A rich source of phytoestrogens, which help some symptoms of the menopause and might protect against certain cancers. Rhubarb is a good source of vitamin C, manganese and potassium, as well as having a mild laxative action. Do not eat the leaves, which are poisonous, and do not cook rhubarb in an aluminium pan (see page 114).

Soya Soya and soy products, such as tofu and miso, are rich sources of phytoestrogens, which give significant protection against coronary heart disease, menopausal symptoms, endometriosis, benign breast disease, fibroids and cancer of the breast or prostate

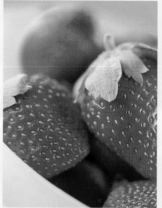

gland. As little as 50 g (2 oz) per day could be enough to provide these benefits. Soy is also a rich source of protein, calcium and fibre.

Strawberries Another fruit containing ellagic acid, a phytochemical that blocks the effects of some cancer-causing chemicals. Weight for weight, strawberries contain one and a half times as much vitamin C as citrus fruits, and are also a good source of iron.

Sweet potatoes These orange-fleshed tubers are a rich source of betacarotene and phytoestrogens, which can help menopausal symptoms and protect against certain cancers. A good source of potassium, vitamin C and fibre.

Tomatoes Containing lycopene, a carotenoid pigment that is a powerful antioxidant, tomatoes protect against coronary heart disease and certain cancers. A good source of betacarotene, potassium and vitamins C and E.

Tea Green tea is a rich source of antioxidants that seem to reduce the risk of certain cancers, especially those of the stomach and bladder. Fermented (black) tea is currently under investigation, as it is thought to retain these beneficial properties. Research suggests that those drinking at least four cups of tea per day are half as likely to have a heart attack as non-tea drinkers, and less likely to suffer from high blood pressure. Tea is a rich source of phytochemicals and the trace element manganese. It is also one of the few natural sources of fluoride, so might protect against tooth decay. When following a detox programme, consider switching from coffee to tea. Although tea contains some caffeine, it is also rich in flavonoids, the chemicals known to give red wine its beneficial properties.

Fibre

Dietary fibre (roughage) aids the digestion and absorption of foods, promotes a healthy bacterial balance and provides important bulk to stimulate the movement of digested food through the intestines. Thanks to its sponge-like action, fibre also assists in the elimination of toxins from the bowel. For every 1 g of fibre you eat, bowel motions increase by an estimated 5 g in weight.

Fibre from different plants varies widely in its composition. Recent research suggests that bowel bacteria adapt to the types of fibre you eat. After a few weeks of eating a fibre-rich diet, they release more of the enzymes needed to break down the different fibre types. This means that fibre reaching your colon is then broken down more quickly so some of the benefits are lost unless you regularly vary the types of fibre you obtain. Eat as wide a range of fibre-rich foods as possible from a variety of wholegrain sources, such as fruit and vegetables. It helps to increase intakes slowly so that you don't develop wind and bloating from an initial fibre overload. It also helps to take a probiotic supplement (see page 45) for improved intestinal health. When following a detox programme, a fibre supplement, such as psyllium husks, is recommended to help scrub and scour the bowel. If choosing to take fibre supplements long term, however, vary the type you take.

Left: *Wholegrains are a major source of fibre*

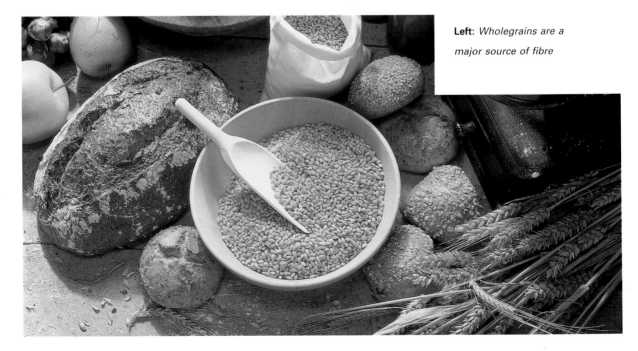

Salt

Although it is probably the most common flavouring on food, salt has little to recommend it in nutritional terms. If trying to follow a balanced diet, bear the following things in mind.

- Avoid obviously salty foods.
- Do not add salt to food during cooking or at the table.
- Where salt is essential, use mineral-rich rock salt rather than table salt, or use a low-sodium brand of salt sparingly.
- Adding lime juice to food stimulates the tastes buds and decreases the amount of salt you need, too.

Note: When food labels quote sodium rather than salt content, the figure needs to be multiplied by 2.5 to give the true salt content. For example, a serving of soup containing 0.4 g sodium contains 1 g salt.

Adaptogenic Supplements

Adaptogens are substances that strengthen, balance and regulate all the body's systems. They have wide-ranging, beneficial actions and boost immunity through several different actions to help you adapt to a wide variety of new or stressful situations. Research suggests that adaptogens work by increasing the production of energy in body cells and by making the uptake of oxygen and processing of cell wastes more efficient. This encourages cell growth and increases cell survival. Many adaptogens have been shown to normalize blood sugar levels, hormone imbalances, disrupted biorhythms and the physical and emotional effects of stress.

Adaptogens seem to work best as an energy stimulant if fatigue is not directly due to excess physical exertion but to an underlying problem such as poor or irregular diet, hormone imbalance, stress or excess consumption of caffeine, nicotine or alcohol. Lifestyle changes to redress the balance (e.g. stopping or cutting back on smoking) are also important to re-energize the body. When adaptogens are used together with vitamin C and the B complex, the effectiveness of the adaptogens are often improved.

When following a balancing detox programme, the usual advice is to take one or more of the following herbal supplements, depending on your needs: ashwagandha (Indian ginseng), astragalus, black cohosh, cat's claw, Chinese and American ginsengs, echinacea, pfaffia (Brazilian ginseng), red clover, reishi, schisandra and Siberian ginseng.

Ashwagandha (Withania somnifera)

This small, evergreen shrub, native to India, the Mediterranean and Middle East, is also known as winter cherry or Indian ginseng. It is used in ayurvedic medicine as a balancing, restorative tonic and adaptogen, which improves resistance to stress. It reduces anxiety and promotes serenity and deep sleep. It is also said to strengthen muscles, tendons and bones, improve concentration, boost immunity and build *ojas* – the primary energy of the body.

Ashwagandha's adaptogenic properties are well researched, and could be superior to ginseng in improving mental acuity, reaction time and physical performance in healthy people. Studies also suggest that it can prevent the depletion of vitamin C and cortisol (an adrenal hormone) in subjects under stress, as well as preventing stress-related gastrointestinal ulcers. Other studies have shown that it can increase haemoglobin levels and has anti-inflammatory properties. Ashwagandha is also renowned as an aphrodisiac. *Dose:* 1–2 g of powdered root per day in capsules standardized to contain 2–5 mg withanolides: 150–300 mg.

As some people find ashwagandha difficult to digest, it is often taken with ginger, warm milk, honey or hot water.

Astragalus (Astragalus membranaceus)

This balancing herb has actions similar to those of Chinese ginseng (see page 82). It is recommended as a tonic for those who are physically active, especially in winter, to increase stamina and endurance. It is said to fortify the constitution and helps to overcome fatigue by increasing feelings of vitality. Astragalus is widely used as a blood cleanser, has a mild diuretic action and promotes sweating. It can also lower blood pressure and encourage a healthy fluid balance. Astragalus is especially helpful to balance and restore normal immune function. *Dose:* 250–500 mg twice a day

Black cohosh (Cimicifuga racemosa)

Also known as squaw root or black snakeroot, black cohosh is a herbaceous perennial native to North America. Insects avoid the plant, which led to its Latin name (*cimex* = bug; *fugere* = to flee). The root and rhizomes are harvested in the autumn and dried for medicinal use.

Black cohosh is an adaptogen known for its ability to help the body adapt to changing situations and valued for its hormone- and mood-balancing properties. It contains a number of oestrogen-like plant hormones (phytoestrogens), and is especially helpful for women with premenstrual, menstrual or menopausal problems. It can reduce moods swings and feelings of depression, anxiety and tension, and is an effective natural alternative to hormone replacement therapy. Since its unique oestrogen action does not stimulate oestrogen-sensitive tumours (and might even inhibit them), black cohosh extracts have been safely given to women with a history of breast cancer.

Dose: 1–2 mg twice per day in capsules standardized to provide 27-deoxyacteine; 0.3–2 ml per day in liquid extract; or 2–4 ml per day in tincture form.

Black cohosh should not be taken during pregnancy or when breast-feeding. Excess amounts can cause headaches behind the eyes, nausea or indigestion.

Cat's claw (Uncaria tomentosa)

Derived from a South American vine, cat's claw has been hailed as the "wonder drug of the botanical kingdom". Its root and bark contain potent alkaloids, some of which have been found to possess anti-cancer, anti-inflammatory and antiviral properties. Cat's claw can balance and support immune function by encouraging white blood cells to absorb and destroy (phagocytose) micro-organisms, abnormal cells and foreign particles. Its extracts contain potent antioxidants and helps to protect against environmental toxins, including the genetic damage caused by ultraviolet light and smoking cigarettes.

Dose: 300 mg per day, taken as two standardized capsules of 150 mg. Gradually build up to 750 mg taken as five 150 mg capsules.

As cat's claw increases the immune rejection of foreign cells, it should not be used during pregnancy, when breast-feeding, by anyone who has recently had – or is scheduled to receive – an organ/bone marrow transplant or skin-graft, or by those taking immunosuppressive drugs. Some researchers also recommend that cat's claw be stopped two days before and two days after receiving chemotherapy.

Chinese and American Ginsengs

Ginsengs belonging to the Panax family of plants have been used in the Orient as revitalizing and balancing tonics for over 7,000 years (see page 82).

Echinacea (Echinacea purpurea)

Purple coneflower, as it is commonly known, is a traditional remedy first used by Native Americans to treat respiratory infections, reduce fever and relieve allergic reactions. It boosts immunity and promotes healing by increasing the number and activity of white blood cells responsible for attacking both viral and bacterial infections. Echinacea has been shown to almost double the length of time between infections compared with those not taking it, and, when infections do occur, they tend to be less severe. It can be used for both prevention and treatment. Echinacea is also detoxifying and encourages elimination by promoting sweating.

Dose: 300 mg dried extract (tablets/capsules) three times per day for 1–2 weeks. It is not usually taken long term for detox.

Below: *Purple coneflower can boost immune function*

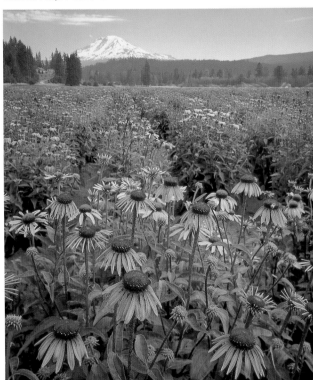

Pfaffia (Pfaffia paniculata)

Also known as suma or Brazilian ginseng, pfaffia is a ground-covering vine native to Brazil. It is regarded as a panacea for all ills, as well as a sustaining food rich in vitamins, minerals and amino acids. Its abundant plant hormones (up to 11 per cent by weight) have oestrogen-like actions and are able to reduce high cholesterol levels.

Although pfaffia is unrelated to Chinese ginseng, it has similar balancing and adaptogenic properties, and can help the immune system adapt to various stresses, including overwork, illness and fatigue. It is used to boost physical, mental and sexual energy levels, as well as producing a general sense of well-being. Its efficacy in treating female hormonal imbalances means that it is widely used as a natural hormone replacement therapy. Pfaffia is also helpful in chronic fatigue syndrome and improves sleep.

Dose: 1 g per day in standardized extracts (capsules) containing 5 per cent ecdysterones.

Pfaffia should not be taken by women with hormone-sensitive conditions, such as pregnancy and certain female cancers, except under specialist advice.

Diabetics should monitor sugar levels closely, as pfaffia seems to boost insulin production, normalizes blood sugar levels and might reduce insulin requirements.

Red clover (Trifolium pratense)

One of over 70 different species of clover native to Europe and Asia, red clover contains three classes of oestrogen-like plant hormones. It is widely used to balance high oestrogen levels because it dilutes the effects of stronger oestrogens in the body, but is also used to boost levels where oestrogen is low. It is therefore commonly prescribed to treat premenstrual syndrome, endometriosis, fibroids and menopausal symptoms.

Dose: 500 mg per day in tablets standardized to contain 40 mg isoflavones.

Do not take during pregnancy or when breast-feeding.

Reishi (Ganoderma lucidum)

One of seven different varieties of *Ganoderma* mushroom, reishi, literally "spiritual mushroom", is regarded as the most superior. The Chinese call it *ling zhi* (mushroom of immortality) and classify it as equal in importance to ginseng.

Reishi has been used medicinally for over 3,000 years as a powerful adaptogen, balancing tonic and antioxidant. It is traditionally used to strengthen the liver, lungs, heart and immune system, to increase intellectual capacity and memory, boost physical and mental energy levels and to promote vitality and longevity. It is now also used to speed convalescence, regulate blood sugar levels and help minimize the side effects of chemotherapy or radiotherapy. It reduces blood-clotting and can lower blood pressure and cholesterol levels.

Reishi helps bring the body's natural functions back to peak performance, enhances energy levels and gives a more restful night's sleep. There is no cross-reaction with traditional button mushrooms, and it can be safely taken by those allergic to field mushrooms.

The effects of reishi are enhanced by vitamin C, which increases absorption of the active components.

Dose: 500 mg capsules 2–3 times per day.

Mild side-effects can occur during the first week of taking reishi. These include diarrhoea (often avoided if the tablets are taken with food), irritability, thirst, dry skin rash or mouth ulcers.

Schisandra (Schisandra chinensis)

This aromatic woody vine, native to northeastern China, is a popular tonic also known as *wu wei zi* (five-flavoured fruit) because it tastes simultaneously salty, sweet, bitter, sour and pungent.

Like ginseng, schisandra has powerful adaptogenic properties that help the body to cope during times of stress. It has been found to increase the oxygen uptake of cells and improves mental clarity, irritability, forgetfulness and prevents emotional and physical fatigue. It is regarded as a calming supplement and also boosts liver function, enhances immunity and heart function, and improves allergic skin conditions such as eczema. Schisandra is traditionally taken for 100 days to boost energy and vitality and produce radiant skin. Perhaps that is why it has a high reputation as an aphrodisiac.

Dose: 250–500 mg capsules 1–3 times per day.

Siberian ginseng (Eleutherococcus senticosus)

From a deciduous, hardy shrub, native to eastern Russia, China, Korea and Japan, comes a root that has similar actions to that of Korean and American ginsengs, but it is not closely related.

Siberian ginseng is one of the most widely researched herbal adaptogens. It is used extensively to improve stamina and strength, particularly during or after illness, and when suffering from other forms of stress and fatigue. Russian research suggests that those taking it regularly have 40 per cent fewer colds, flu and other infections than those not taking it, and take a third fewer days off work due to health problems. Little wonder, then, that Siberian ginseng is taken by 20 million Russians every day to improve performance, wellbeing and adaptation to stress or change.

Siberian ginseng is also used to counter jetlag, and has been shown to help normalize high blood pressure and raised blood sugar levels. It is particularly popular with athletes, as it can significantly improve performance and reaction times by as much as a quarter.

Dose: 1–2 g per day in capsules standardized to contain more than 1 per cent eleutherosides; occasionally up to 6g per day is recommended when there is severe stress or reduced immunity present. It is traditionally taken for 2–3 weeks followed by a two-week break for those who are generally young, healthy and fit. Those who are older, weaker or unwell can take their doses continuously. Take on an empty stomach unless you find it too relaxing, in which case take it with meals.

Do not use (except under medical advice) if you suffer from high blood pressure, a tendency to nosebleeds, heavy periods, insomnia, rapid heart beat (tachycardia), high fever or congestive heart failure. Do not take during pregnancy or when breast-feeding, except under specific medical advice.

Balancing Complementery Therapies

A number of complementary therapies can be used for their balancing actions during detox. These include acupuncture,

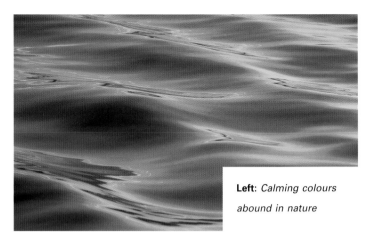

Left: *Calming colours abound in nature*

the Alexander technique, chiropractic, colour therapy, cranial osteopathy, crystal therapy, cymatics, homeopathy, naturopathy, osteopathy, reiki and spiritual healing.

Acupuncture

The ancient Chinese practice of acupuncture can be used to balance the flow of life-force energy in the body and is a useful complementary therapy during the detox process.

Alexander technique

Based on the belief that poor posture and faulty body movements contribute to ill health, the Alexander technique (AT) uses gentle exercises and movements to teach you how to stand and move correctly without undue stress. As well as improving physical coordination, AT has a holistic approach that addresses mental and emotional wellbeing. By improving the ways of thinking and focusing attention on how tasks are performed, it also helps to reduce stress and conserve energy.

Many of the symptoms associated with toxicity can be helped by learning AT. It is especially helpful for stress-related problems as it teaches you how to release tension and remain relaxed.

Chiropractic

This therapy is based on a belief that poor body alignment and abnormal nerve functioning are direct causes of ill health. Practitioners have a finely tuned sense of touch and use their hands to manipulate the spine with rapid, direct, yet gentle thrusts to realign muscles, tendons, ligaments and joints. These strengthen and balance the body's nerve supply, correct poor alignment, ease tension and promote relaxation. The key to the success of these adjustments is in the speed, dexterity and accuracy with which they are performed.

McTimoney chiropractic is a variation in which joints other than the spine are manipulated. It also includes gentle fingertip manipulation.

Colour therapy

Every colour vibrates at its own frequency, as does every living thing, including all the cells in the body. Colour therapy taps into this, using the energy of lightwaves to balance and heal. As a result, colour can effect your emotions and wellbeing.

A colour therapist uses colour vibrations to correct imbalances in the energy vibrations of cells to restore wellness during your detox programme. Shades of blue, for example, are restful, help to lower blood pressure and improve sleep, while magenta, the colour of "letting go", is used in small amounts to help free you from certain toxic thoughts. Green is the calming colour of nature and represents freshness, regeneration and growth: it is an especially good colour to wear during detox as it helps to neutralize stress and nervous tension, and releases repressed emotions and fears.

Natural sunlight contains all colours of the spectrum – red orange, yellow, green, blue, indigo and violet – so it bathes us in a sea of colour, although this is only obvious when light is split with a prism or atmospheric water to create a rainbow.

Your Aura

Everyone is surrounded by an aura of energy, which is made up of seven influences or chakras. Each chakra contains the full spectrum of colour, but a single colour is dominant in each one. Different coloured lights or crystals may be used to clear the chakra with which it is associated.

Red:	The root chakra, at the base of the spine
Orange:	The sacral chakra, in the pelvis
Yellow:	The solar plexus chakra, below the sternum
Green:	The heart chakra
Blue/Turquoise:	The throat chakra
Indigo:	The brow chakra
Violet:	The crown chakra

Most therapists use a colour together with its complement (the colour that is opposite and balancing in its qualities and effects). You might be asked, for example, to choose three out of eight coloured cards to reveal your current emotional and physical state. These colours might be used along with their complementary colours to help balance your vibrational health. This could involve having coloured lights beamed on to your body, being encouraged to visualize certain colours, and being advised on which colours to wear and which coloured foods/juices to consume. White should be worn underneath therapeutically coloured clothes to filter out unwanted colour vibrations.

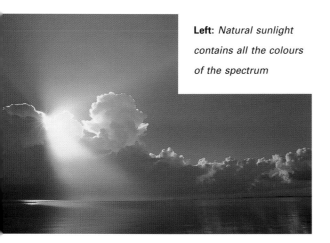

Left: *Natural sunlight contains all the colours of the spectrum*

Seeing complementary colours

A colour's balancing vibration can easily be seen by staring at a particular colour for a while, then closing your eyes. The complementary colour will appear as an after-image on the inside of your eyelids:

Green is neutral

Blue complements red

Yellow complements violet

Orange complements indigo

Cranial osteopathy and Craniosacral therapy

Cranial osteopathy involves manipulating the slight flexibility between the joints of the skull to improve the circulation of fluid, blood and lymph in the head. Lymph is tissue fluid that having bathed body cells, is drained away via the lymphatic system of vessels. Practitioners believe that the cerebrospinal fluid that nourishes the brain and spinal cord pulsates at 6–15 times per minute, and that these pulsations (known as the cranial rhythmic impulse) affect every cell in the body due to the continuity of fluids and tissues. Cranial osteopathy balances the inner movements and tensions inside you to relieve a range of problems such as headache, insomnia, low mood and digestive disorders.

Craniosacral therapy is a similar balancing treatment that involves the gentle laying on of hands and manipulation of both the skull and spine.

Crystal therapy

This treatment balances the body by using the energy derived from crystals. Clear quartz, for example, allows all colours of the spectrum to pass through it, while coloured quartz absorbs and reflects certain wavelengths of light due to minute traces of impurities such as iron (amethyst) or manganese/ titanium (rose quartz). Crystals resonate at their own individual frequency and can receive, store and transmit energy. When pressure is applied to a quartz crystal, this energy is given off in the form of an electric current – the basis of their use in electronics. Crystals help to ground and heal you by balancing and restoring energy levels. Kirlian photography (see page 17) reveals that every crystal has its own energy aura. When this interacts with a person's aura, it is believed to absorb negative vibrations, restore balance and re-energize.

In general, it is important to select crystals that you are particularly drawn to because

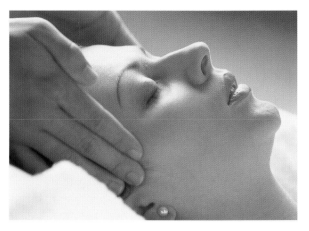

Above: *Cranial osteopathy can relieve tension*

they will be the appropriate ones to help balance your current problem. You can also choose particular types of crystal that are known to help heal particular symptoms. As in colour therapy (see page 67), different coloured crystals are associated with each of the seven energy centres (chakras) in the body.

Cymatics

A balancing complementary therapy based on the fact that every cell in the human body is surrounded by an electromagnetic energy field. This resonates at its own

COLOUR	CHAKRA	CRYSTAL	EFFECT
Red	Root	e.g. ruby, garnet	Calming, balances stress and tension
Orange	Sacral	e.g. carnelian	Activates emotions and encourages openness and release
Yellow	Solar plexus	e.g. citrine, tiger's eye, topaz	Strengthens vitality and releases repressed emotions
Green	Heart	e.g. emerald, jade	Encourages inner peace, self-acceptance and love; balances hormones
Blue	Throat	e.g. aquamarine, turquoise	Encourages self-expression
Indigo	Brow	e.g. blue sapphire, lapis lazuli	Strengthens intuition and heightens awareness; calming and relaxing
Violet	Crown	e.g. amethyst	Deeply calming and relaxing; balances insomnia, headache, stress, anxiety and fear

individual frequency. In health, cells vibrate together in harmony, but if these harmonious relationships become disrupted, imbalances and ill health will result. In cymatics, healing soundwaves are passed through the body to restore and reinforce those frequencies that are normally associated with health and wellbeing. The therapy can help many problems, including stress, anxiety, depression, high blood pressure, muscle and joint pains.

Homoeopathy

A balancing therapy that overcomes imbalances by treating like with like (see page 47).

Naturopathy

Based on the belief that the body can balance and heal itself, given the right conditions, naturopathy aims to identify the underlying cause of illness rather than merely relieving the symptoms. A naturopath will focus on maintaining a balance between the body's biochemistry, its structure and the emotions, and might recommend a variety of treatment options, including dietary changes, vitamins, minerals, biochemic tissue salts, herbal remedies, hydrotherapy, massage, homoeopathy, reflexology, relaxation techniques and sometimes manipulation. Many naturopaths are also trained in homoeopathy, herbalism, iridology, osteopathy, chiropractic or psychotherapy. They encourage a healthy lifestyle, with plenty of fresh air, relaxation and sleep, adequate mineral water intake, reduced exposure to pollution and a positive mental attitude. Skin brushing, water sprays and friction rubs are often recommended to stimulate skin function and to boost the circulation.

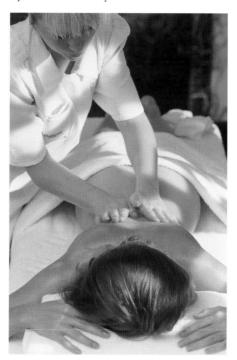

The dietary approaches used are cleansing and balancing, with a wholefood, high fibre and preferably organic diet, concentrating on fresh foods that are as raw as possible. A naturopathic diet is low in salt and fat, high in fibre and antioxidants, and contains plenty of nuts, seeds, grains and pulses for protein.

If you wish to follow a detox programme under professional supervision, a naturopath can guide you.

Osteopathy

A balancing therapy based on the mechanical structure of the body, osteopathy involves gentle manipulation of the joints and soft tissues to correct poor alignment, relax muscles, improve body function and restore health. Correcting these things helps to restore the body's ability to heal itself. The manipulation ranges from gentle massage to sudden, swift mobilizations of joints. Osteopathy can help a wide range of problems, including aches and pains, headache, dizziness, constipation and abdominal discomfort.

Reiki

A natural method of healing, reiki balances mind, body and spirit. The practitioner places his or her hands in a series of positions on the fully clothed body to channel and transmit the energy of the universal life-force. Reiki speeds up the vibrating energy so that it can resonate in a state of wellness. By balancing the vibrational state, physical and emotional equilibrium is attained.

Spiritual healing

Sometimes known as hands-on healing or faith healing, spiritual healing is a therapy that channels balancing and healing energy into you. The healer is the channel for the energy rather than the sources, which is believed to be of a divine nature. However, you do not have to be a believer in order to receive and benefit from the power of spiritual healing. The energy that is transferred from the healer helps to balance the body's own natural repair processes which have become depleted.

Above: *Many healing techniques involve the laying on of hands*

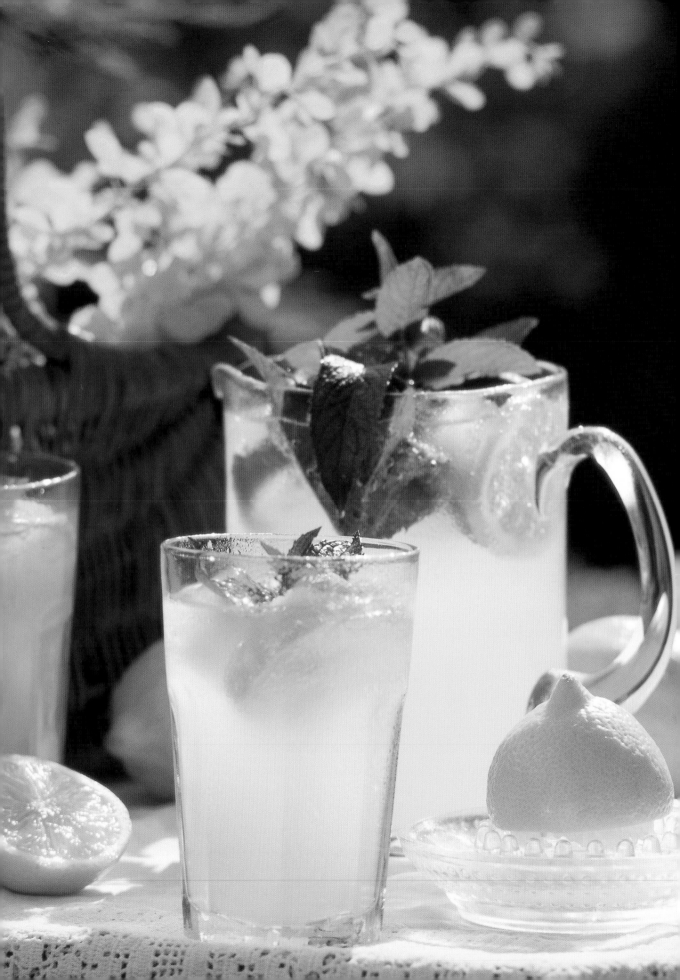

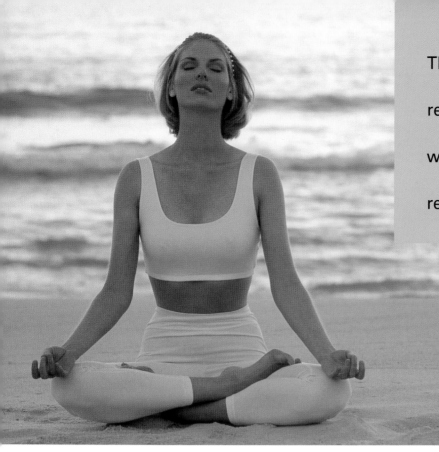

The new found energy released during detox will help you feel more refreshed than before. Enhance this process by eliminating sources of stress.

Refresh

Detox will refresh your body and bring a new sense of vitality. To help this process, take steps to reduce any stress in your life, and make use of aromatherapy oils and refreshing supplements.

Reduce stress

Stress is one of the main factors that drags you down, and you will not feel fully refreshed until you have dealt with the sources of it in your life. Stress is a term used to describe the symptoms produced when you are under excessive pressure. A certain amount of stress is necessary to meet life's challenges, but too much is harmful and can leave you feeling tired, irritable and tense. The symptoms of stress result from high levels of circulating stress hormones, such as

adrenaline, which literally put your systems into a state of "red alert". This results in blood sugar levels rising to provide energy; bowels emptying to make you lighter for running; pupils dilating to help you see better; respiratory rate going up so that more oxygen enters your circulation; pulse and blood pressure increasing so that more oxygen and nutrients flow to important organs and tissues; and the circulation decreasing to some parts of your body (e.g. the gut) so that more blood can be diverted to the muscles.

These effects were designed to help primitive man survive by putting him into the appropriate physical state to fight or flee from dangerous animals. Nowadays, you rarely need to fight or flee, and the effects of stress build up inside you rather than getting burned off through a sudden burst of physical activity. This means that your body stays on red alert, leading to physical and emotional symptoms of stress.

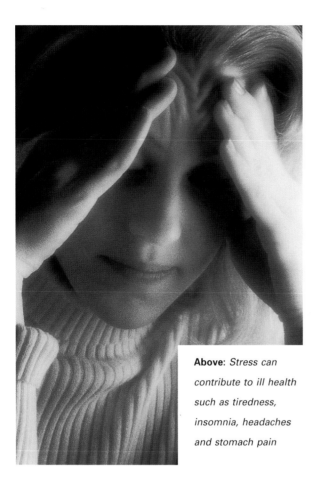

Above: *Stress can contribute to ill health such as tiredness, insomnia, headaches and stomach pain*

Emotional

- Loss of concentration
- Inability to make decisions
- Forgetfulness
- Over-defensiveness
- Overwhelming feelings of anxiety and panic
- Fear of rejection
- Fear of failure
- Feelings of guilt and shame
- Negative thoughts
- Moodiness
- Extreme anger
- Loss of sex drive and sexual problems
- Obsessive or compulsive behaviour
- Feelings of isolation
- A feeling of impending doom

Behavioural Symptoms of Stress

Stress also leads to a number of behavioural traits that are, in themselves, potentially toxic. These can include:

- Compulsive eating habits
- Excessive use of alcohol or tobacco
- Abuse of drugs
- Avoidance of places or situations
- Increased aggression
- Change in sleeping habits, particularly early wakening

SYMPTOMS OF STRESS
Physical

- Tiredness
- Sweating
- Flushing
- Nausea
- Insomnia
- Palpitations
- Rapid pulse
- Dizziness
- Faintness
- Trembling
- Pins and needles
- Numbness
- Headache
- Chest pain
- Stomach pain
- Diarrhoea
- Period problems

Stress is a highly toxic state that lowers immunity and is associated with an increased risk of illness, including infections, eczema, psoriasis, depression, high blood pressure, heart attack, stroke and even cancer. The two main sources of stress that you need to address during a detox programme are internal and external.

Sources of internal stress depend on personality type and can include tiredness, physical unfitness and disruption of biorhythms, perhaps from shift work or jetlag. Being unsure of your aims in life, feeling unable to cope with situations and having a negative self-image are also potent causes of stress.

Sources of external stress are related mainly to change, particularly if change is imposed on you. It causes uncertainty, which induces anxiety and this triggers stress. External changes can come from all aspects of your life, including family, social relationships, lifestyle and work.

One of the best ways to identify sources of stress in your life is to keep a stress diary. This involves writing down everything that makes you feel stressed, noting how you respond and how you remedy the situation to help stop the stress returning.

Try to fill in your diary immediately after each stressful event – don't leave it until later or you will not remember exactly how you felt.

At the end of a week go back over your diary and try to identify the main sources of stress, how much control you have over them, and the steps you can take to reduce their effects. Think about your habits and consider whether any are making things worse. For example, rather than shopping on a Friday evening when the supermarket is busy, consider shopping at a quieter time, and investigate having essential groceries delivered, perhaps from a local organic box scheme.

Date: Friday, 10 June

Time	Situation	Feelings	Response	Future Remedy
8.30	Overslept	Dreadful	No breakfast	Set back-up alarm
9.30	Late for work	Anxious	Drove too fast	Negotiate flexi-time?
15.00	Stuck in traffic on way to important meeting	Frustrated; developed tension headache	Listened to classical music	Leave in plenty of time
18.00	Supermarket crowded	Hot and flustered	Rushed out, forgetting to buy some things	shop when store quieter. Unwound with a glass of wine and aromatherapy bath

Steps to controlling stress

1. Work out what makes you stressed and change those that can be changed.
2. Set yourself realistic goals and tackle big problems one step at a time.
3. Make decisions calmly, not under pressure of deadlines.
4. Learn to be patient, talk more slowly and listen without interrupting.
5. Change your perceptions of a stressful situation and view it in perspective.
6. Be assertive: say no when appropriate, and mean it; don't let yourself be put upon and overloaded with tasks.
7. Think more positively to improve self-esteem and self-confidence.
8. Improve your ability to cope – detox will help enormously.
9. Change your behaviour.
10. Put aside relaxation time every day for a quiet read, a candlelit aromatherapy bath, or just to close your eyes and rest (see Chapter 7).

Tips to stop stress in its tracks

- Stop what you are doing and inwardly say "Calm" to yourself.
- Take a deep breath in and let it out slowly.
- Shake your hands and arms briskly, then shrug your shoulders.
- Go for a brisk walk to boost circulation to your brain.
- Go somewhere private and groan or shout as loudly as you can.
- Place a few drops of Bach Rescue Remedy under your tongue.
- Listen to calming background music to help you unwind.
- Practise the Chinese inner smile exercise (see page 74).

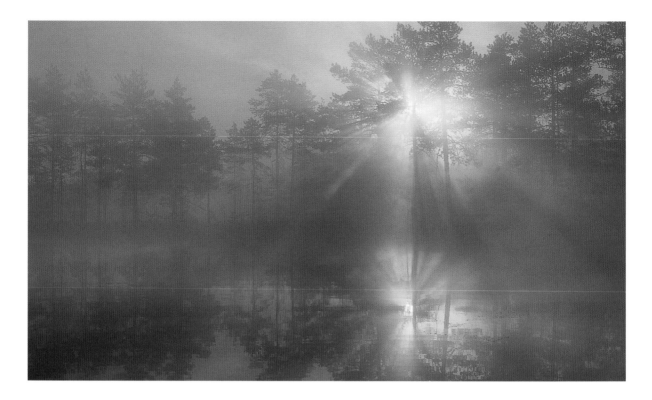

Chinese Inner Smile

A quick and refreshing exercise is a Chinese technique called the inner smile. It takes only a few minutes and brings rapid relaxation and rejuvenation to help leave tensions behind.

1. Sit comfortably with your back straight and your arms relaxed at your side.
2. Imagine something that makes you smile.
3. Allow yourself to smile internally so that it is felt only by you – the smile does not have to be visible to anyone else.
4. Let the smile shine out of your eyes and travel inwards to spread all over your body, before concentrating just below your navel in an area known to the Chinese as *tan tien* (the seat of your constitutional essence).
5. As the smile radiates within, notice how relaxed, calm and refreshed you feel.
6. Once you feel relaxed yet energized, you can continue what you were previously doing enriched by feelings of warmth, harmony and inner strength.

If returning to work after completing this exercise, ensure that you find time for frequent breaks. Take a couple of minutes every hour to walk about or stretch.

Refreshing Breathing Exercises

Stress can change your breathing pattern, leading to hyperventilation, when you take quick, irregular, shallow breaths. As a result, you inhale too much oxygen and exhale too much carbon dioxide, making your blood excessively alkaline. This leads to symptoms of dizziness, faintness and pins and needles (often around the mouth) and can trigger a panic attack. Use the following exercises to refresh your breathing in situations where you feel stressed:

1. Sit back in your chair.
2. Drop and widen your shoulders by moving your arms.
3. Expand your chest and fill your lungs as far as possible.
4. Breathe in and out as deeply as you can, being aware of the rise and fall of your abdomen rather than your chest. Repeat five times without holding your breath.
5. Continue to breathe regularly, getting your rhythm right by counting 1–3 when breathing in, and 1–4 on breathing out.

Above: *The Chinese inner smile will leave you feeling relaxed, calm and refreshed*

When Panic Rises

Use this exercise to refresh your sense of control when you feel panic rising:

1. As panic wells up, quietly say STOP to yourself.
2. Breathe out deeply, then breathe in slowly.
3. Hold this breath for a count of three and breathe out gently, letting the tension go.
4. Continue to breathe regularly, imagining a candle in front of your face. As you breathe, the flame should flicker but not go out.
5. Continue breathing gently, and consciously try to relax. Let your tense muscles unwind and try to speak and move more slowly.

Exercises to Relieve Stress

Try the following exercises to refresh yourself regularly throughout the day, or as a general energizing boost at the end of a long day.

Arm swings

1. Stand up and take a few deep breaths.
2. Stretch both arms in front of you at shoulder height.
3. Let your arms relax and drop to your sides, letting them swing to a standstill. Repeat several times.
4. Finally, raise your arms above your shoulders and swing energetically.

Hand shakes

1. Shake each hand and arm in turn for a minute or two.
2. When you stop, your muscles will feel soft and relaxed.
3. Repeat, using your legs and feet if you wish.

Neck relaxer

1. Imagine you are carrying a heavy weight in each hand so that your shoulders are pulled towards the floor.
2. Drop the weight and feel the tension release. Repeat several times and feel your neck become less tense.

Shoulder circles

1. Circle your left shoulder in a backward direction five times. Repeat with the right shoulder.
2. Circle your left shoulder in a forward direction five times. Repeat with right shoulder.
3. Circle both shoulders forward five times, and then backwards five times.

Leg shakes

1. Balance on one leg, supporting yourself against a wall or chair if necessary.
2. Shake the weight-free leg in the air a few times, and circle your foot at the ankle joint.
3. Repeat with the opposite leg.

Refreshing aromatherapy oils

Aromatherapy uses aromatic essential oils produced by special glands in the leaves, stems, bark, flowers, roots or seeds of certain plants. These oils contain many active ingredients in a highly concentrated and potent form, which, because they are volatile,

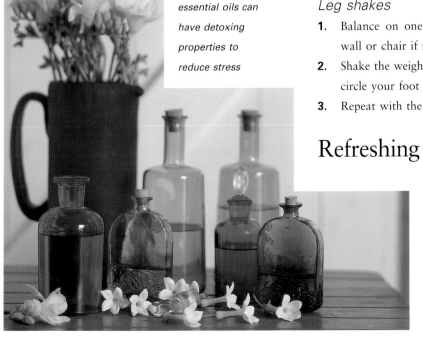

Left: *Aromatherapy essential oils can have detoxing properties to reduce stress*

readily evaporate to release their powerful scent. Essential oils are highly concentrated and, with a few exceptions, should always be diluted with a carrier oil (see below) before coming into contact with the skin.

Preparing Your Own Essential Oils

Essential oils should never be used in their concentrated form. At the very least add 1 drop of essential oil to 5ml (1 medicinal teaspoon) of carrier oil (e.g. avocado, calendula, grapeseed, jojoba, sunflower or wheatgerm) to make a 1 per cent solution. For larger quantities, the dilutions are as follows:

10 drops essential oil to 100 ml (3 ½ fl oz) carrier oil = 0.5% solution

20 drops essential oil to 100 ml (3 ½ fl oz) carrier oil = 1% solution

40 drops essential oil to 100 ml (3 ½ fl oz) carrier oil = 2% solution

During the day, aromatherapy oils can be inhaled to freshen your mind and improve clarity during the detox process. It is important to use natural rather than synthetic oils, and select those that have been grown organically. Natural oils generally have a fuller, sweeter aroma, which provides a greater therapeutic benefit. Similarly, 100 per cent pure essential oils – while more expensive – are desirable, as they have not been mixed with alcohol or other additives.

Oils to match your mood

To refresh, try black pepper, geranium, ginger, grapefruit, lemon balm, peppermint or sandalwood.
To improve clarity of thought, try basil or cardamom.
To increase concentration, try lemon.

Refreshing Supplements

A number of supplements are used for their ability to refresh. These include fo-ti, ginger, ginkgo, St John's wort, phosphatidyl serine and thiamine.

Fo-ti (Polygonum multiflorum)

A perennial climber native to central and southern China, fo-ti is one of the oldest Chinese tonic herbs. It is famous for its rejuvenating and revitalizing properties, and is taken by millions of men and women in the East as a general restorative and aphrodisiac. It is also used to reduce the premature greying of hair.
Dose: 5 g per day in tablet form. (Fo-ti is often taken with ginseng.)

Ginger (Zingiber officinale)

The warming, refreshing action of ginger is described on page 46.

Ginkgo (Ginkgo biloba)

The maidenhair tree, from which gingko is derived, is one of the oldest known plant species on Earth and is often described as a living fossil. Gingko is one of the most popular health supplements in Europe and can improve memory and concentration, as well as increasing peripheral blood flow. It is also helpful for stress-induced anxiety, depression and migraine.
Dose: 120 mg per day taken as capsules standardized to contain at least 24 per cent ginkolides. The stimulating effects last 3–6 hours, but might not be noticed until after 10 days' treatment.

St John's Wort (Hypericum perforatum)

This remedy has been used for over 2,000 years to improve emotional wellbeing. It is an effective and gentle anti-depressant, found to help in at least 67 per cent of those with mild to moderate depression. Studies involving over 5,000 patients show that its effects begin to be felt within two weeks of starting the course, the optimum effect being reached within six weeks. In the same study 82 per cent of patients also suffered less irritability, anxiety, hot flushes, sweating and disturbed sleep. Low sex drive – a common accompaniment to stress and depression – improved in 60 per cent of people within three months.
Dose: 300 mg three times a day in extracts standardized to contain 0.3 per cent hypericin. Best taken with food.

Side effects are significantly less likely than with prescription antidepressants: 1 per cent of patients reported indigestion, allergic reactions, restlessness and tiredness. Do not take during pregnancy, when breast-feeding or in combination with other antidepressants, except under medical supervision. It is best to avoid alcohol and direct exposure to sunlight, especially if fair-skinned. If you are taking prescribed medicines check with your practitioner before using.

Phosphatidyl serine

This chemical plays an important role in the way brain cells communicate with each other. When taken as a supplement, it helps to improve brain function and memory, especially in those aged over 50.

Dose: 500–1500mg capsules or tablets phospholipid complex daily.

Thiamine

Also known as vitamin B1, thiamine is water soluble and plays an important role in metabolism and nerve cell function. It is essential for the production of energy from glucose, and for healthy brain cells. Thiamine has a refreshing effect on mood, helping you feel calmer, more agreeable, clear-headed, elated and energetic. People with low levels of thiamine (usually those aged over 55) tend to lack self-confidence and often suffer from depression. Supplements can help to increase feelings of general wellbeing, improve fatigue and boost appetite.

Common causes of thiamine deficiency include drinking large amounts of coffee or tea (which

destroy the vitamin), stress (which quickly uses up available thiamine stores) and drinking too much alcohol (which interferes with thiamine metabolism).

Dose: 1.4 mg per day. Any excess is readily lost in the urine.

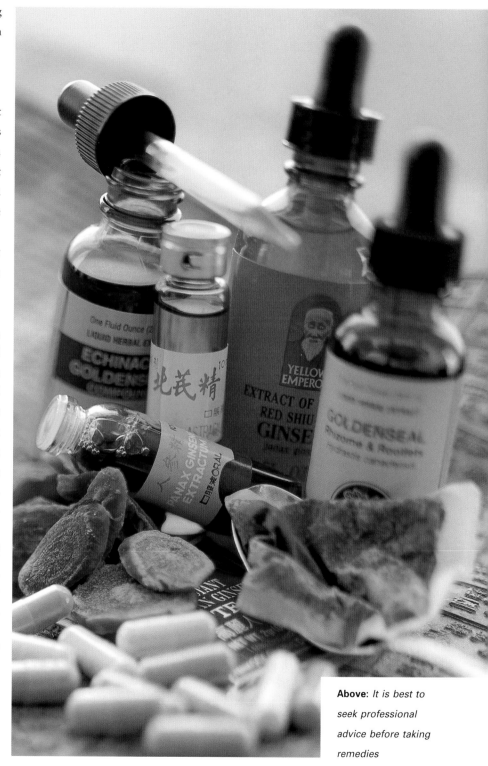

Above: *It is best to seek professional advice before taking remedies*

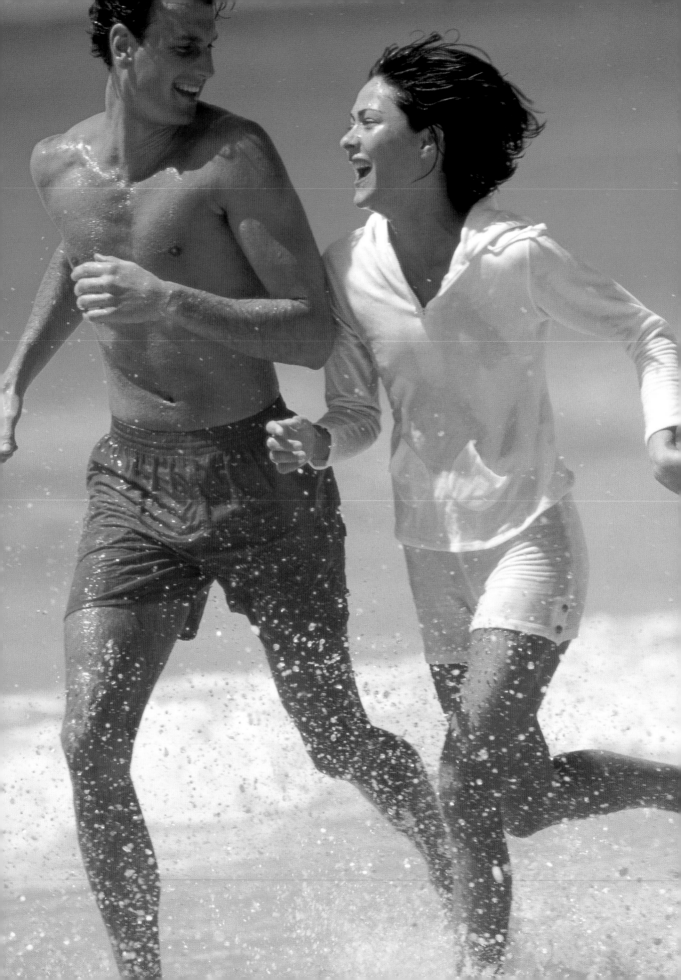

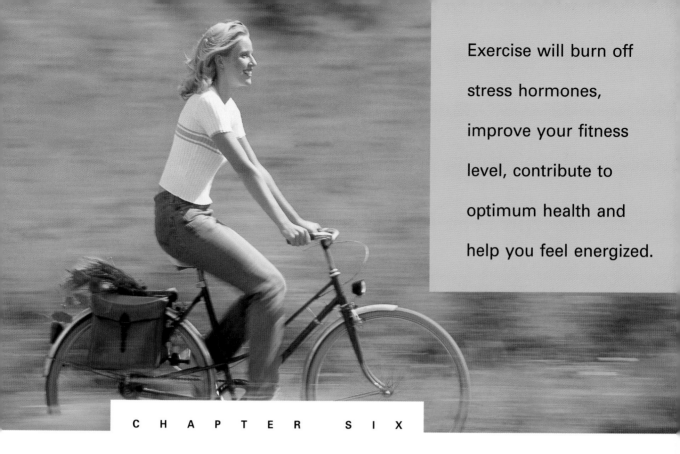

Exercise will burn off stress hormones, improve your fitness level, contribute to optimum health and help you feel energized.

Energize

Exercise is an important supplement to the detox process, as it promotes the mobilization of toxins stored in fat cells, and increases their excretion through sweat glands in the skin. By contrast, lack of exercise leads to a sluggish metabolism and venous congestion, which is a build up of fluid in the veins which can contribute to varicose veins, or leak out into tissues to cause swollen ankles, promoting the build up of toxins.

While following a strict juice and fruit diet, do only gentle exercise, such as walking or cycling. Once you are eating a healthy, balancing diet, however, aim to exercise to the point of perspiring as often as possible, and at least for 15–30 minutes five times a week. Joining a gym is one of the most popular ways to become fit, as qualified instructors are available to tailor individual fitness regimes to your particular needs.

Do it yourself

If you are serious about detox but not sure you want to join a gym, various items of exercise equipment can be purchased for use at home. Although they might seem expensive, when compared to the monthly costs of using a gym, they can be good value. Whatever you choose to do, the financial outlay provides a great incentive for exercising regularly.

Some of the most popular forms of detox home exercises are described below, along with the benefits they provide for strength, stamina and suppleness:

✳ = Slight effect

✳✳ = Beneficial effect

✳✳✳ = Very good effect

✳✳✳✳ = Excellent effect

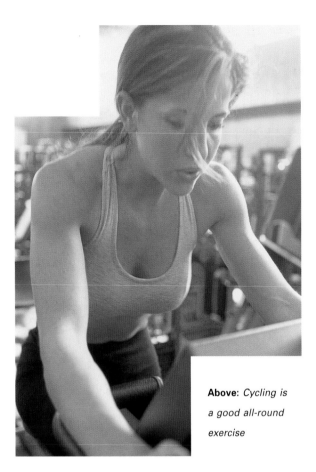

Above: *Cycling is a good all-round exercise*

Speedropes

Widely used by athletes as part of their training regime, speedropes combine a traditional aerobics work-out with a specially designed skipping rope for burning off calories. They are great fun, but quickly make you realize how unfit you are. An easy detox exercise to carry anywhere.

Strength ✳✳   *Stamina* ✳✳✳   *Suppleness* ✳✳

Step Systems

A video of low-impact aerobics that involve stepping on and off a low step. The best steps can be safely adjusted to various heights, but don't go too high, as this increases the risk of lower leg injuries, particularly to the Achilles' tendon. Research shows that the optimal height for a step aerobics work-out is 15 cm (6 in).

Strength ✳✳   *Stamina* ✳✳✳   *Suppleness* ✳✳✳

Trampolines

Personal trampolines, or bouncers, are a fun way to get fit after your detox programme, but are even better when used with *Starbound* (see page 127). This book gives you lots of exercises to perform on the bouncer and allows you to tailor the work-out to your individual needs.

Strength ✳✳   *Stamina* ✳✳✳   *Suppleness* ✳✳✳

AB Trainers

Abdominal muscle trainers are more effective than normal abdominal crunches that you might do in the gym. It is a hoop of metal with attached cushions on which you lie and rock to and fro. The AB trainer isolates the abdominal muscles and gives them a full work-out, while supporting the head and neck and eliminating strain on the lower back. Great for those with middle-aged spread in the spare-tyre area.

Strength ✳✳✳✳   (abdominal muscles only)

Stamina ✳✳   *Suppleness* ✳

Rowing machines

Rowing is a popular form of home exercise, giving a good, all-round, low-impact aerobic work-out. Excellent for muscle tone throughout the body, especially the legs and abdominals. Vigorous rowing uses as many calories as running at a rate of 11 km (7 miles) per hour.

Strength ✳✳   *Stamina* ✳✳✳   *Suppleness* ✳

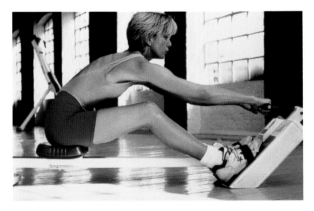

Above: *Rowing is excellent for general muscle tone*

Recumbent exercise bicycles

These machines have elevated pedals, so they are driven by leg power rather than leg weight and gravity as on more upright bicycles. The recumbent position and cushioned seat also relieve stresses and strains on the lower back and guarantee that you won't get saddle-sore. A video display on the machine offers a variety of courses and effort levels.

Strength ✳✳   *Stamina* ✳✳✳✳   *Suppleness* ✳✳

Health riders

A cross between an exercise bike and rowing machine, with a bucking-bronco action. Health riders use your own weight to provide resistance, so you can increase your workload by using different foot settings and raising the front end of the machine. Although they exercise just about every muscle in the body, the machines do not leave you aching next day, as little stress is placed on the muscles and joints.

Strength ✳✳✳✳   *Stamina* ✳✳✳✳

Suppleness ✳✳✳✳

Cross-country ski exercisers

Ski exercisers, which mimic the actions of cross-country skiing, claim to be the world's most efficient form of aerobic exercise. They work both your arms and legs, burning up 35 per cent more calories than a step regime. They offer an excellent all-round work-out at different resistances – on the flat or uphill. As a bonus, they are low impact, so they do not jar the joints.

Strength ✳✳✳✳   *Stamina* ✳✳✳✳

Suppleness ✳✳✳✳

Treadmills

One of the best ways to walk briskly or jog during winter months. A treadmill gives you your own indoor running track, allowing you to start off at a brisk walk and slowly increase your speed to suit your progress. You can listen to music or watch TV, and don't have to worry about the weather or safety at night.

Strength ✳✳ (brisk walk)   ✳✳ (jogging)

Stamina ✳✳✳ (brisk walk)   ✳✳✳✳ (jogging)

Suppleness ✳ (brisk walk)   ✳✳ (jogging)

Elliptical-cross trainer

Claims to give you the equivalent of a 25-minute workout on a treadmill or cycle in just 15 minutes. This revolutionary piece of gym equipment is one of the most popular items in clubs, and a version can now be bought for home use. It suspends your body on pedals, so you run/walk/step/cycle in mid-air. As your feet are not slamming into the floor as you run, it is kind on the joints. Upper body resistance is provided by arm-poles that work with an elliptical motion, ensuring a high-energy body workout for maximum calorie burning and detox. Some 40 per cent more gluteal activity – exercising the buttock muscle – occurs on elliptical machines than on standard treadmills, and 30 per cent more than on a climber. Your work-out can be as rigorous or moderate as you choose.

Strength ✳✳✳✳   *Stamina* ✳✳✳✳   *Suppleness* ✳✳✳✳

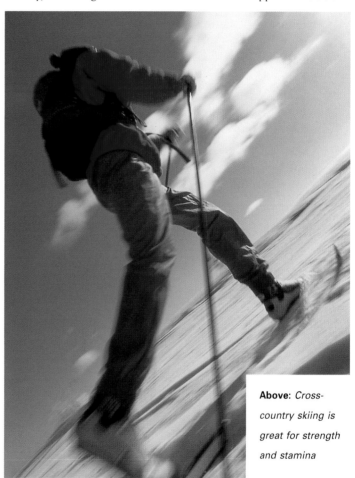

Above: *Cross-country skiing is great for strength and stamina*

Energizing supplements

Detox tends to have an energizing effect, but there are times when you might feel you need an extra boost. Among the supplements that can help are Chinese and American ginsengs, guarana, maca, yerba maté, royal jelly, bee pollen, propolis, B group vitamins, iron, magnesium, CoQ10 and NADH.

Ginseng

Ginseng comes from the Panax family of plants. *P. quinquefolium*, usually referred to as Chinese, Korean or Asian ginseng, is a perennial plant native to those countries from which it takes its common names, but is now rare in the wild. High quality ginseng is collected in the autumn from cultivated plants that are five or six years old. White ginseng is produced by air-drying the root, while red ginseng (which is more potent and stimulating) is produced by first steaming and then drying the root. The closely

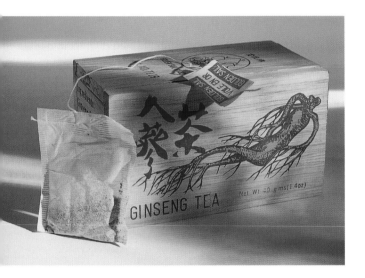

related *P. quinquefolius,* from the woodlands of east and central North America, is commonly known as American ginseng and has a similar action. Preferred by some for its sweeter taste and gentler effect, it is thought to have more *yin* (heat-reducing capacity) than Chinese ginseng. American ginseng is said to be best for relieving fatigue caused by nervous conditions, anxiety and insomnia, while Chinese/Korean ginseng is better for fatigue with general weakness and loss of energy.

Ginseng has been used in the Orient as a revitalizing, energizing and balancing tonic for over 7,000 years. Clinical trials have confirmed that it helps the body adapt to physical or emotional stress and fatigue. It is stimulating and restorative, improving physical and mental energy, stamina, strength, alertness and concentration. It has a normalizing effect on hormone imbalances, boosts the metabolic rate and is also reputed to be an aphrodisiac. *Dose:* 200 mg per day to start, building to an optimal dose of 600 mg. American ginseng should contain at least 5

per cent ginsenosides, while Korean ginseng should contain 15 per cent. In the East, ginseng is taken two weeks on, two weeks off. It should not be taken for more than six weeks without a break.

Buy only good-quality ginseng from a reputable company, as cheap versions sometimes contain very little active ingredient.

Do not take ginseng if you have high blood pressure or an oestrogen-dependent condition, such as pregnancy, or cancer of the breast, ovaries or uterus, as it contains oestrogenic compounds.

Guarana (Paullinia cupana)

Guarana is a Brazilian bush that is probably the best-known herbal medicine from the rainforest. Its dried seeds contain a complex of natural stimulants, including guaranine, which is similar to caffeine, and saponins, similar to those found in Korean and American ginseng. Natives refer to guarana as the food of the gods and use its sun-dried seeds to make a sweet, cola-like, energizing tonic.

Guarana increases physical, mental and sexual energy levels and relieves fatigue. It is less likely to produce the irritability, poor sleep and tremor linked with excess caffeine intake, as the guaranine is buffered by oily saponins, which produce a natural timed-release effect. Although energizing, it also has a calming effect and does not usually interfere with sleep or make stress-related symptoms worse.

Research in Denmark has found that volunteers who took guarana extracts for three months had a significant increase in energy levels and reacted better to stress. In Japan, doctors advise long-distance lorry drivers to chew guarana gum to stay awake behind the wheel, and, as a result, the number of accidents due to drivers falling asleep has significantly decreased. Guarana also seems to boost the immune system, thin the blood, reduce fluid retention, decrease appetite and raise the metabolic rate. It relieves tension headache, premenstrual syndrome and period pains.

During a detox programme, guarana is best used as a substitute for those who find it difficult to reduce their caffeine intake.

Dose: 1 g per day in the form of capsules, a wine-based elixir, energy bars, chewing gum or an energy drink. A single dose provides an energy boost lasting up to six hours. Choose products that have been sun-dried and ground as roasting converts more guaranine to caffeine.

People sensitive to the effects of guarana respond to it in the same way as caffeine, so use it sparingly at first while you assess the way you respond to it.

Note: Guarana is a restricted substance in certain sports.

Maca (Lepidium meyenii)

Maca is a root vegetable related to the potato and grows in the Peruvian Andes at heights of around over 4,000 metres (12,000 ft). It is a good source of carbohydrate, amino acids, fatty acids, vitamins B1, B2, B12, C and E, plus the minerals calcium, phosphorus, zinc, magnesium, copper and iron, which is perhaps why it has been used as a food staple since before the time of the Incas. Its tubers contain a number of plant hormones that increase energy and stamina. Some researchers believe that maca is superior to red Korean ginseng, and it is sometimes referred to as Peruvian ginseng.

Dose: 1 g capsules or tablets 2–3 times per day.

Yerba maté (Ilex paraguariensis)

Derived from a tree that grows in the rainforests of Paraguay, yerba maté leaves are made into a tea that is rich in nutrients, especially vitamin C. The leaves also contain xanthine alkaloids related to those found in coffee and guarana, which increase mental alertness and acuity without the caffeine side effects of nervousness or sleep disturbance. It can even improve sleep patterns by normalizing the amount of time spent in rapid eye movement (REM) sleep and deep, delta-wave sleep, giving a deeper, more refreshing rest. In fact, some users find that they actually need less sleep than usual when taking maté.

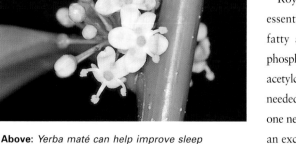

Above: *Yerba maté can help improve sleep*

Maté is used mainly as an energizing tonic to boost vitality and overcome physical exhaustion or mental fatigue, especially during times of stress. It stimulates the adrenal glands to boost production of corticosteroids and is therefore classed as an adaptogen, helping the body to adapt and cope with stressful times. It is a popular indigestion remedy, a mild diuretic and improves constipation by both softening hard faeces and gently stimulating bowel movements. By helping the elimination of wastes and toxins through both bowels and kidneys, it is a useful detoxifying agent.

Maté's calming effects relieve anxiety, poor concentration and nervousness. It also acts as a substitute for alcohol, and helps liver regeneration, especially when trying to reduce alcohol intake.

During a detox programme, yerba maté is best used as a substitute for those who find it difficult to reduce their caffeine or alcohol intake.

Dose: 2–3 infusions per day.

Note: As yerba maté contains high quantities of tannins, it is best not to consume it with meals as it can impair the absorption of nutrients.

Royal Jelly

Also known as bee's milk, royal jelly is a milky white substance secreted in the salivary glands of worker bees. It is a highly concentrated food given to all bee larvae for the first three days of their lives. After that, they're nourished on a diet of honey, pollen and water, except for the larva that is destined to become a queen bee. She continues to receive royal jelly to stimulate and sustain her development. As a result, the queen bee grows 50 per cent larger than other genetically identical female bees and has a lifespan nearly 40 times longer.

Royal jelly is a rich source of essential amino acids, essential fatty acids, sugars, sterols and phosphorus compounds, as well as acetylcholine – a neurotransmitter needed to transmit messages from one nerve cell to another. It is also an excellent source of vitamin B5 (pantothenic acid).

While royal jelly is traditionally taken as an energizing tonic, to prolong youthfulness and to improve the complexion, it also seems to alleviate anxiety, sleeplessness and memory loss, boost the immune system and is widely reputed to be an aphrodisiac. It needs to be blended with honey (or powdered in capsules) to preserve the active ingredients during storage.

Dose: 50–100 mg per day taken on an empty stomach. **Note:** Do not take royal jelly if you are allergic to bee products.

Bee Pollen

Bee pollen is an ultra-fine dust made up of sex cells produced on the anthers of male flowers.

Above: *Royal jelly is a great pick-me-up*

Bees collect the pollen when foraging for nectar and store it in the hive as food for young bees. Bee pollen is a nourishing food, rich in amino acids, carbohydrates, fatty acids, vitamins, minerals and trace elements. The ancient Romans and Greeks considered bee pollen an energizing food, so it was probably an ingredient of ambrosia – the secret food of the gods, which guaranteed eternal life. Like so many energizing products, bee pollen is widely reputed to act as an aphrodisiac.

Dose: 250mg – 2g per day for at least one month. **Note:** Do not take if you are allergic to bee products or pollen.

Propolis

This natural bee antiseptic is secreted to maintain hygiene in the hive. It contains antioxidants and is a rich source of B group vitamins, which might explain its reputation as an energy-boosting supplement. It is also taken to increase immunity, especially in winter months. Around 1 per cent of people taking it develop a mild allergic skin reaction, so start with a low dose to see how it suits you. *Dose*: 250–500 mg tablets or capsules per day.

B group vitamins

B1, B2, B3, B5, B6, B12 and folic acid are involved in a wide variety of metabolic reactions needed to produce energy in the body.

Vitamin B1, also known as thiamine, is essential for the production of energy from blood sugar (glucose) and for the synthesis of some amino acids.

Vitamin B2 (riboflavin) plays an important role in metabolizing proteins, fats and carbohydrate to produce energy, and as it cannot be stored in the body, regular dietary intakes are essential.

Vitamin B3 (niacin) plays an important role in metabolism and enzyme function, and is essential for releasing energy from muscle sugar stores (glycogen) and for the uptake and use of oxygen in cells. As niacin is important for the processing of fatty acids released from body-fat stores, it is used medicinally to lower abnormally high cholesterol and triglyceride levels. It also combines with the mineral chromium to form the body's glucose tolerance factor (GTF). This is essential for the action of insulin, which controls the way glucose is taken up into body cells.

Vitamin B5 (pantothenic acid) is vital for many energy-yielding metabolic reactions involving carbohydrates, fats and protein. It is also necessary for making glucose and fatty acids in the liver, both being important fuels for muscle cells. It is therefore thought to boost energy reserves and improve athletic performance. It plays a role in the production of adrenal gland hormones during times of stress and in maintaining a healthy nervous system. It has also been suggested that vitamin B5 supplements might be useful during detox. By ensuring that fatty acids released from body-fat stores are fully broken down, it can reduce the formation of ketones (see page 24), so hunger pangs and weakness are reduced.

Vitamin B6 (pyridoxine) is essential for the proper functioning of over 60 enzymes. It is needed for the synthesis of genetic material, amino acids and proteins, and for metabolizing body stores of carbohydrate (glycogen) and essential fatty acids.

Recent research provides preliminary evidence that people with chronic fatigue syndrome are lacking in certain B group vitamins. Taking energizing vitamin B complex supplements might therefore help to overcome long-term tiredness.

Dose: 50–100 mg per day vitamin B complex in divided doses.

Iron

Iron is an essential mineral, the two main forms of which are ferrous and ferric. It is the ferrous form that is absorbed by the body, and is needed for the production of haemoglobin, the red blood pigment that transports oxygen and carbon dioxide around the body. Iron is also found in a protein called myoglobin, which binds oxygen in muscle cells for ready access during exercise. Lack of iron leads to anaemia and fatigue.

Many enzyme systems rely on iron for optimum function, including those involved in the production of energy from carbohydrate, fat and protein.

Iron supplements given alone can decrease the absorption of zinc and other essential minerals, such as manganese, chromium and selenium, so it is usually combined with other minerals and trace elements.

Vitamin C taken at the same time as iron-rich foods or supplements helps to boost iron absorption by keeping it in the ferrous form.

Dose: 15 mg per day maximum, unless you have proven iron deficiency. Excess iron can cause constipation or indigestion and is also toxic.

Magnesium

A metal responsible for the function of over 300 enzymes, magnesium is also vital for every major metabolic reaction in the body, from the synthesis of proteins, essential fatty acids and genetic material to the production of energy from glucose. Few enzymes can work without it and lack of magnesium leads to cell death due to the depletion of energy stores. Magnesium levels decrease with age, and lack of magnesium might play a role in premature ageing by reducing efficacy of enzymes and metabolic reactions.

Dose: 300 mg per day. Included in vitamin and mineral tablets and capsules

Co-enzyme Q10

Also known as ubiquinone or CoQ10, co-enzyme Q10 is a vitamin-like compound that improves energy levels and endurance, strengthens the pumping action of the heart and also acts as an antioxidant. It is needed by cells to process oxygen and generate energy-rich molecules. CoQ10 is made in the liver (from the amino acid phenylalanine) and is found in almost every type of food, including meat, fish, wholegrains, nuts and green vegetables. Body levels of CoQ10 start to decrease in those aged over 20, however, as dietary sources are absorbed less efficiently from the intestines and its production in the liver starts to fall. Low levels of CoQ10 mean that cells do not receive all the energy they need, so they function sub-optimally and are more likely to become diseased or even die. CoQ10 is useful during detox as it reduces the risk of gum infection and inflammation. It is especially helpful for those over 40 who are suffering from fatigue. To get maximum benefit, it should be taken with adequate amounts of B and C vitamins.

Dose: 30–90 mg per day. Intakes of up to 180 mg are recommended for general use by some researchers. It usually takes three weeks, and occasionally up to three months, before energy levels are noticeably increased.

NADH

A substance involved in energy production in cells. Some people have found it helpful for improving fatigue and concentration, but there is little experience in its use at present.

Energizing Aromatherapy Oils

The following essential oils are used for their uplifting and energizing qualities. Use them to scent a room, or place a few drops on a handkerchief and inhale at regular intervals.

- Basil
- Black pepper
- Eucalyptus
- Geranium
- Peppermint
- Rosemary

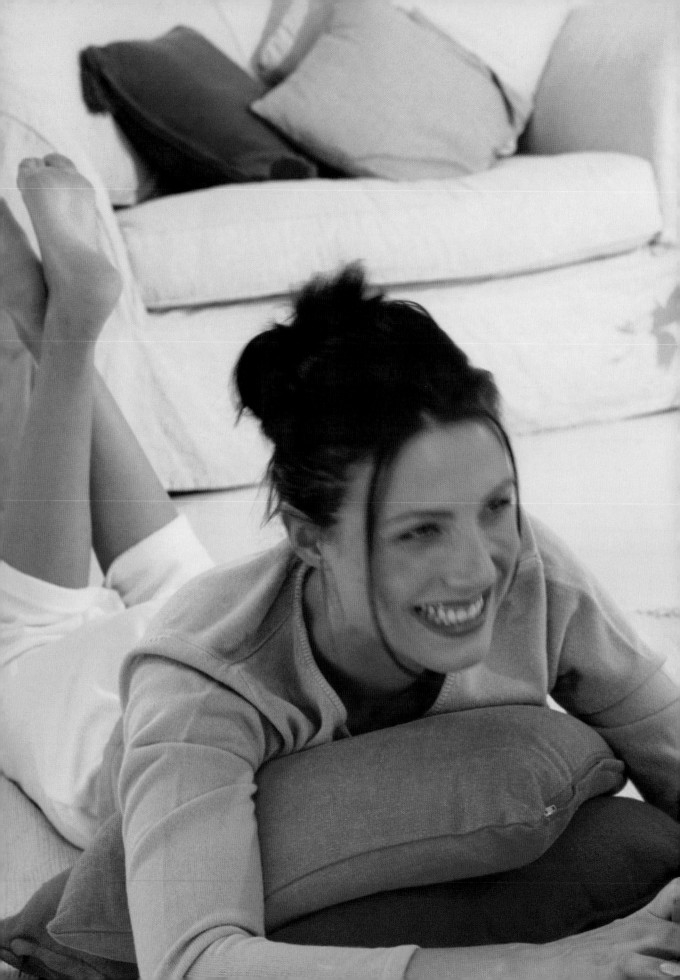

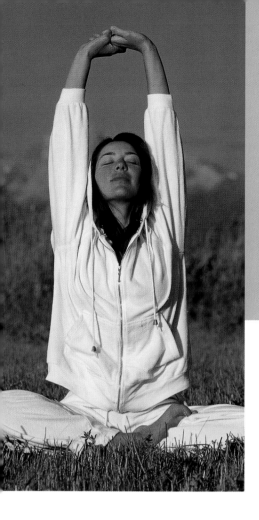

It is important to balance exercise with periods of rest and relaxation. However, if you lead a hectic and stressful lifestyle, it can be difficult to learn the art of unwinding.

Relax

Relaxation is an important part of the detox process and has beneficial effects on mind and spirit, as well on the physical body. A few relaxation exercises combined with a candlelit aromatherapy bath will help you to wind down the day towards a refreshing night's sleep. A number of complementary therapies revolve around the importance of relaxation and meditation. When your mind and body need a little extra help, a number of gentle relaxing herbs are available, too.

Deep relaxation

For a deep relaxation exercise that works on different muscle groups to relieve tension, set aside at least half an hour. This exercise is especially beneficial after a long soak in a warm, aromatherapy bath.

1. Find somewhere quiet and warm to lie down. Remove your shoes and wear loose, lightweight clothing. Close your eyes and keep them closed throughout the session.

2. Lift your forearms into the air, bending them at the elbow. Clench your fists hard and concentrate on the tension in these muscles.

3. Breathe in deeply and slowly. As you breathe out, start to relax and let the tension in your arms drain away. Release your clenched fists and lower your arms gently down beside you. Feel the tension flow out of them until your fingers start to tingle. Your arms might feel as though they don't belong to you. Keep breathing gently and slowly.

4. Now tense your shoulders and neck, shrugging your shoulders up as high as you can. Feel the tension in your head, shoulders, neck and chest. Hold it for a moment. Then, slowly let the tension flow away, breathing gently and slowly as it does so.

5. Now lift your head up and push it forwards. Feel the tension in your neck. Tighten all your facial muscles. Clench your teeth, frown and screw up your eyes. Feel the tension on your face, the tightness in your skin and jaw, the wrinkles on your brow. Hold this tension for a few seconds, then start to relax. Let go gradually, concentrating on each set of muscles as they relax. A feeling of warmth will spread across your head as the tension is released. Your head will feel heavy and very relaxed.

6. Continue in this way, working next on your back muscles (provided you don't have a back problem). Pull your shoulders and head backwards and arch your back upwards. Hold this for a few moments before letting your weight sink comfortably down as you relax. Check that your arms, head and neck are still relaxed, too.

7. Pull in your abdomen as tightly as you can. Then, as you breathe out, slowly release the tension and feel it drain away. Now push out your stomach, as if tensing against a blow. Hold this tension for a few moments, then slowly relax.

8. Make sure tension has not crept back into the parts of your body you have already relaxed. Your upper body should feel heavy, calm and relaxed.

9. Now, concentrate on your legs. Pull your toes up towards you and feel the tightness down the front of your legs. Push your toes away from you and feel the tightness spread up your legs. Hold this position for a few moments, then lift your legs into the air, either together or one at a time. Hold for a few moments, then lower your legs until they are at rest.

10. Relax your thighs, buttocks, calves and feet. Let them flop under their own weight and relax. Feel the tension flow down your legs and out through your toes. Feel your legs become heavy and relaxed. Your toes might tingle.

11. Your whole body should now feel very heavy and very relaxed. Breathe calmly and slowly and feel all that tension drain away.

12. Now imagine you are lying on a warm, tropical beach with the waves gently lapping on the shore. Relax for at

least 20 minutes, occasionally checking your body for tension. In your own time bring the session to a close.

Sleep well

A good night's sleep is vital for health. When you wake up feeling refreshed, you are ready to tackle anything that comes your way. When sleep is non-refreshing, though, it can ruin your whole day. The following tips will help you to enjoy a good night's sleep:

✧ Take regular brisk exercise during the day, but not late in the evening, which can keep you awake.
✧ When following a detox programme, try going to bed earlier than normal to give your body extra refreshment.
✧ Take time to unwind from the stresses of the day before going to bed: read a book, listen to soothing music or have a candlelit aromatherapy bath.
✧ Get into the habit of going to bed at a regular time each night and getting up at the same time each morning.

Below: *Relax and unwind in an aromatherapy bath with a good book*

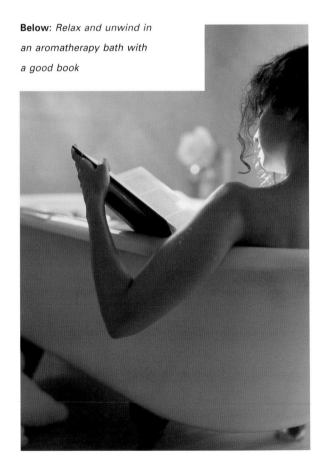

✧ Make sure your bed is comfortable and that your bedroom is warm, dark and quiet.

✧ Sprinkle a few drops of sleep-inducing essential oils on to a handkerchief and tuck it under your pillow.

✧ If you can't sleep, try practising the sequence of relaxation exercises on page 86 so that your whole body feels as if it has melted into the bed.

Relaxing essential oils

- Bergamot
- Benzoin
- Camomile
- Cedarwood
- Clary sage
- Jasmine
- Juniper berry
- Lavender
- Mandarin
- Marjoram
- Neroli
- Nutmeg
- Orange
- Pettigrain
- Rose
- Sandalwood
- Vanilla
- Vettiver
- Ylang-ylang

Relaxing herbal supplements

A number of herbal supplements have a natural sedative action to promote a good night's sleep without unwanted side effects. These include hops, kava kava, lemon balm, oats, passionflower and valerian.

Note: Do not take a supplement containing these herbs if you are taking prescribed sleeping tablets, suffer from marked depression, are pregnant or breast-feeding. They can also cause mild drowsiness, which could affect your ability to drive or operate machinery.

Hops (Humulus lupulus)

Hops have a powerful relaxant effect on the central nervous system and are widely used to ease tension and anxiety and overcome insomnia. They are also used to relieve restlessness, headache and indigestion, which can be signs that you need to detox. Hops are often combined with valerian and lemon balm to promote a good night's sleep.

Dose: 300–400 mg herbal extracts in tablet/capsule.form.

Kava kava (Piper methysticum)

A Polynesian perennial plant, kava has heart-shaped leaves and a massive rootstock that can weigh as much as 10 kg (22 lb). Its botanical name means "intoxicating pepper" and refers to a 3,000-year-old native custom of fermenting fresh kava roots to make a potent alcoholic drink. This is used during a variety of rituals to induce relaxation and mild euphoria, and to enhance dreams. Supplements made from the dried root are not intoxicating, however, although a few people find that they can produce a pleasant, dream-like state.

Kava is widely used to combat mild anxiety, as it is non-addictive and promotes feelings of relaxation and calm. It is mildly sedative, relieves muscle tension and can improve memory and reaction time. Effects are usually noticeable within a week and improvements continue over the next month.

Unlike tranquillizer drugs, kava does not impair driving skills, coordination, or visual perception and judgement at therapeutic doses. Exceeding recommended doses can, however, cause problems.

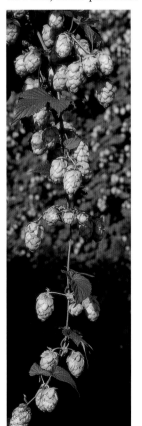

Dose: 100 mg three times per day in products standardized to contain 70 per cent kava lactones.

Note: Some kava teas can provide over 200 mg kava lactones per cup, so do not over-indulge.

Exceeding the recommended dose can cause a variety of side effects and can also adversely affect liver function. Do not combine kava with alcohol, tranquillizers, or illegal drugs, and do not take during pregnancy or when breast-feeding. It should also be avoided by people with Parkinson's disease.

Left: *Hops are useful to help promote a restful night's sleep*

Lemon balm (Melissa officinalis)

Used since ancient times as a healing, soothing herb with calming properties, lemon balm is often combined with valerian to reduce stress and promote sleep.

Dose: 300–600 mg per day

Note: Do not take lemon balm if you are already using prescribed sleeping tablets, are pregnant or breast-feeding. Side effects can include mild drowsiness, which could affect your ability to drive or operate machinery.

Oats (Avena sativa)

Extracts from the young, whole plant or unripe grain, also known as oat straw or wild oats, are widely used as a restorative nerve tonic. Oat straw has a calming effect and is used to help reduce cravings when giving up cigarettes.

Dose: 1 dropperful fluid extract or tincture 2–3 times per day.

People who suffer from coeliac disease (sensitivity to gluten) should allow the tincture to settle, then decant the clear liquid for use.

Passionflower (Passiflora incarnata)

The sedative, analgesic action of this plant reduces stress and encourages natural, restful sleep. Passiflora is used for treating insomnia, anxiety, stress and nervousness, and is often included in herbal tea blends designed to be taken before going to sleep.

Dose: 150–300 mg per day.

Valerian (Valeriana officinalis)

One of the most calming sedative herbs available, valerian helps to reduce feelings of stress, anxiety and tension and induce relaxation and sleep. It is also helpful in overcoming mild depression. Do not take if already using prescribed sleeping tablets.

Dose: 200–300 mg per day. The leaves are usually blended with other herbs.

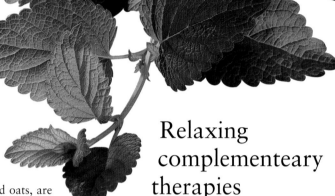

Relaxing complementeary therapies

A number of complementary therapies are used to help induce relaxation. These include autogenic training, flotation, massage, meditation, qigong, tai chi chu'uan and yoga.

Autogenic Training

Autogenic training is a relaxation technique involving the use of passive concentration – when you empty your mind and listen to nothing – and mental exercises to reduce stress and restore physical equilibrium. Once learned, these techniques can be used to obtain almost instant calmness and relaxation. Exercises involve allowing different parts of the body to feel heavy and warm, followed by concentration on the heartbeat and breathing rhythms.

Flotation therapy

As its name suggests, flotation therapy involves lying in a lightproof, sound-insulated tank containing a shallow pool of saline kept at body temperature. The flotation tank screens out light and sound to remove virtually all external stimulation. This allows the floater to enter a profoundly relaxed state in which the brain generates theta waves, which are associated with meditation, creative thought and feelings of serenity. Studies show that the brain continues to produce large amounts of theta waves for up to three weeks after a float.

An additional benefit of flotation is that during detox it reduces the secretion of anti-diuretic hormones. This means that any retained fluid is lost because larger quantities of urine are expelled shortly after a float.

You can obtain a similar deep relaxation in your own bath using mineral salts from the Dead Sea (available from larger health food stores and pharmacies).

Massage

Massage forms the basis of many complementary therapies, including acupressure, aromatherapy and shiatsu. It stimulates the soft tissues of the body and is useful in detox as it encourages the drainage and removal of toxins. Massage is also relaxing and can relieve anxiety, tension and aches and pains, as well as lifting mild depression and improving sleep.

Meditation

Meditation uses the power of the mind to empty itself of thoughts, calm the body and achieve a state of heightened mental or spiritual awareness. By focusing your mind on a particular object or vision, you can screen out distractions and induce a state of profound relaxation and serenity. There are several types of meditation, each of which favours a different technique. This might involve focusing on your breathing rhythm, a universal sound, such as "om", a word or phrase with personal meaning (mantra), a physical object, such as a flickering candle, or an image. Some techniques, such as t'ai chi ch'uan, involve repetitive movements, while others might involve feeling objects, such as pebbles or worry beads.

Transcendental meditation (TM) was developed to fit into the busy, modern way of life. Practised for 15–20 minutes twice a day, TM uses a variety of Sanskrit mantras, which are repeated silently to still the thoughts and find a deeper level of consciousness. This helps to achieve deep relaxation, while maintaining full alertness. It leaves you feeling refreshed mentally and physically, with a mind that is calmer and able to think more clearly.

Qigong

Qigong and the related medical therapy buqi are forms of Chinese yoga that combine meditation and posture to achieve relaxation and breath control. Qigong also helps to channel energy and calm the mind. The basic postures are easy to learn and, unlike tai chi, can be performed in any order.

Tai chi chu'uan

Usually known simply as tai chi, this therapy is sometimes described as meditation in motion. It combines slow, graceful movements with meditation and breathing techniques to calm the mind and improve the flow of the life energy force, *qi*.

The short form of tai chi uses 24 slow movements and postures that flow effortlessly into each other and can be performed in 5–10 minutes. The long form, consisting of 108 movements, takes 20–40 minutes to complete.

Yoga

Although many types of yoga exist, all forms of it combine postural exercises, breathing techniques and meditation to achieve relaxation. Indeed, breath control is considered most important as it embodies the life force, *prana*, to help achieve emotional and mental harmony. This is particularly important during detox.

Left: *Massage and the laying on of hands are widely practised complementary techniques*

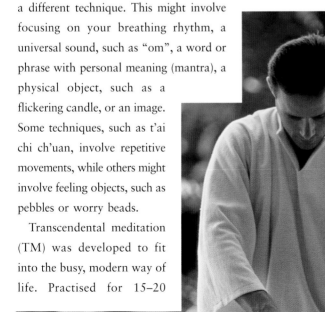

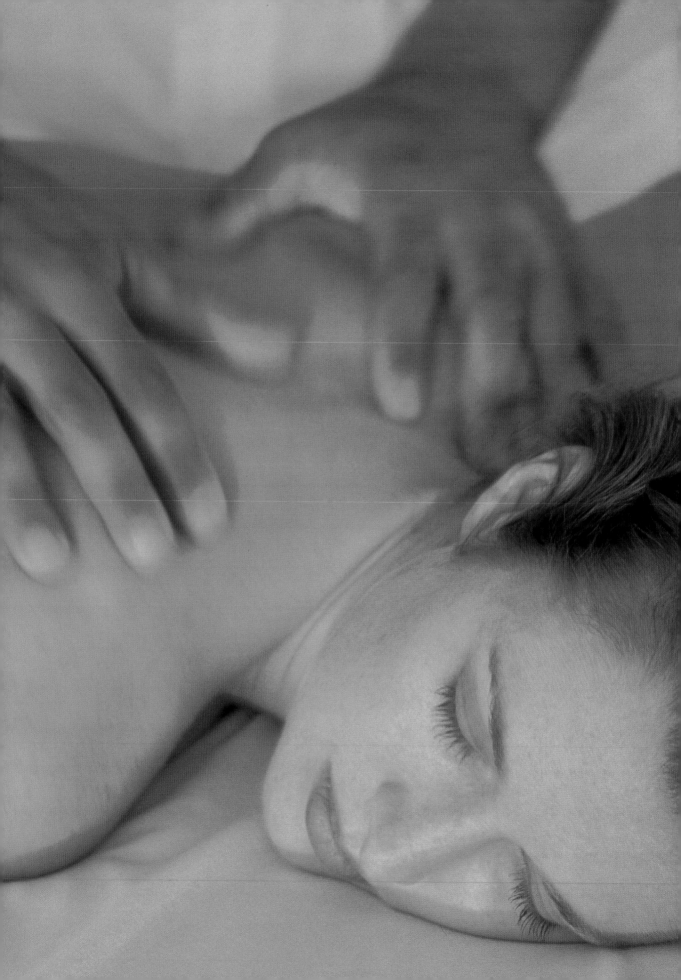

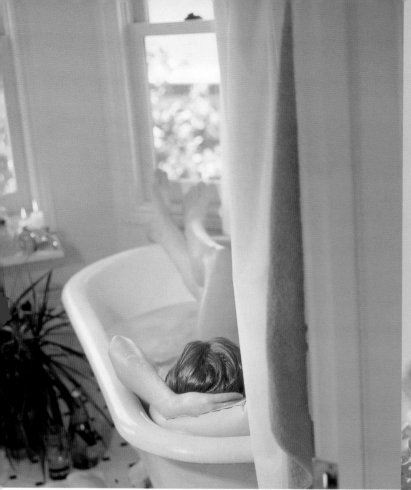

The detox process should be one of enjoyment. So learn to indulge your new self – you deserve it!

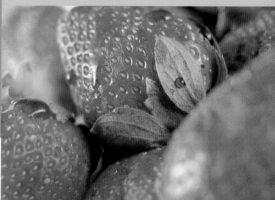

Indulge

Detox should be an enjoyable process. Allow yourself a daily treat, such as a massage, a facial, a quiet hour reading, or a relaxing, candlelit aromatherapy bath. Even putting clean, freshly-ironed sheets on your bed can count as an indulgence after a soothing bath.

If you can make time for a few days away at the end of your detox programme, all the better. You could choose a romantic weekend break with your partner, or a visit a spa or health farm to continue with detox treatments and ultra-healthy foods.

Sweat it out

Therapies that promote perspiration help to sweat toxins out of the body, providing a deep cleansing and stimulating effect. During detox, try to sweat for 15–30 minutes several times a week, or even daily if you can, both through exercise and the application of warmth and steam. A number of useful detox therapies that can also be considered as indulgences include facials, hydrotherapy, steam treatments, saunas, Dead Sea mineral salt soaks and aromatherapy massages.

Quick indulgences

- Soak your feet in a bowl of warm water to which you've added a handful of Dead Sea mineral salts and a few drops of your favourite aromatherapy oil or perfume.
- Add a deep-penetrating conditioning treatment to your hair, wrap it in cling-film and leave to be absorbed while you soak yourself in the bath.
- Buy a CD of birdsong (see Resources, page 126) and lie on your bed listening to the sounds of nature.
- Go to bed an hour earlier than usual and catch up on your reading.
- Exfoliate your body of dead skin cells and the toxins they contain. This can be done in the bath simply by rubbing the skin with a handful of oats, Dead Sea mineral salts, Epsom salts, a natural loofah, or an agave fibre washcloth.
- Apply a luxurious body lotion after bathing and exfoliating – preferably one that is as natural, organic and non-toxic as possible.

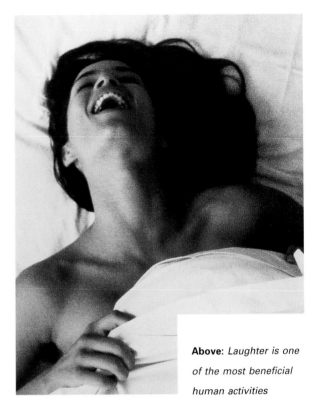

Above: *Laughter is one of the most beneficial human activities*

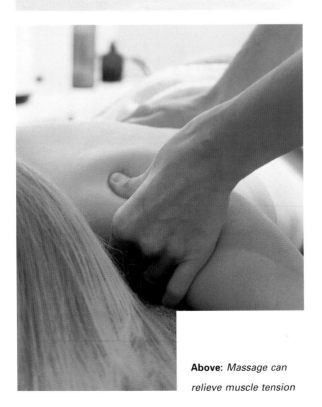

Above: *Massage can relieve muscle tension*

Aromatherapy massage

Massage is a pleasant way of helping to release toxins from fatty tissues under the skin, relaxing tense muscles and easing stress. You and your partner can easily learn to massage each other, thus adding a new dimension to your detox experience.

Massage your partner for 30 minutes, then relax while he or she reciprocates. The following are the secrets of success:

1. Make sure the room is warm with gentle light and slow, relaxing background music.

2. Choose a firm surface to work on: the floor is fine, but spread several towels on it first.

3. Warm the massage oil or lotion by placing the bottle in a bowl of comfortably hot water. Alternatively, rub some oil in your hands to warm it before using.

4. Ask your partner to lie on his or her front, then cover with a large bath towel. Expose the area you are working on, then re-cover it before moving on to the next.

5. Begin with long, flowing, simple strokes that follow the body contours in order to warm the skin. Then vary the pressure and length of stroke you use, keeping the movements flowing and rhythmic, with one hand in contact with the body at all times. Try alternating firm movements with feathery ones. If you find a muscle that seems knotted or tense, concentrate on that area with gentle kneading movements.

When you have finished massaging the back, ask your partner to turn over so that you can work on the front.

6. Massage each arm and leg, keeping the rest of the body covered in the warm towels.

In general, use hand movements that stroke towards the heart, and finish by holding the feet for a few seconds as this helps to "ground" the body.

AROMATHERAPY OILS AND THEIR USES

OIL	CLEANSING	BALANCING	REFRESHING	ENERGIZING	RELAXING
Angelica		✳	✳		
Basil	✳	✳	✳	✳	
Bergamot	✳	✳			✳
Benzoin	✳	✳	✳		✳
Bergamot	✳	✳			✳
Black pepper			✳	✳	
Cardamom			✳		
Camomile	✳	✳			✳
Cedarwood	✳				✳
Clary sage		✳			✳
Coriander		✳	✳		
Eucalyptus	✳	✳		✳	
Fennel	✳	✳			
Geranium	✳	✳		✳	
Ginger		✳			
Grapefruit		✳	✳		
Jasmine		✳			✳
Juniper berry	✳				✳
Lavender	✳	✳			✳
Lemon	✳	✳	✳		✳
Marjoram	✳				✳
Neroli	✳	✳			✳
Nutmeg					✳
Orange		✳	✳		✳
Patchouli		✳			✳
Pettigrain		✳			✳
Peppermint	✳		✳	✳	
Pine		✳	✳		
Rose	✳	✳			✳
Rosemary	✳		✳	✳	
Rosewood		✳	✳		
Sandalwood	✳		✳		✳
Tea tree	✳	✳			✳
Vanilla		✳			✳
Vetiver		✳			✳
Ylang-ylang		✳			✳

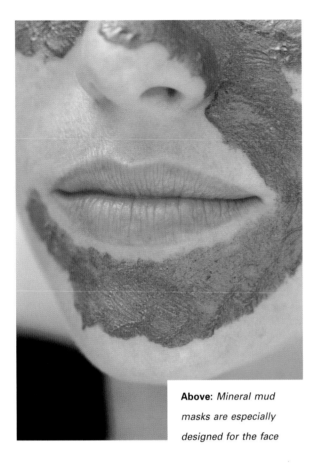

Above: *Mineral mud masks are especially designed for the face*

Dead Sea mineral salt treatments

Ever since the days of Cleopatra, the rich mineral salts and mud derived from the inland sea between Israel and Jordan have been renowned for their beautifying, healing and detoxifying properties. At 400 metres (1,200 feet) below sea level, the Dead Sea is the lowest place on Earth. Over thousands of years, rainwater has trickled down through the rocks and soils of the Jordan Rift Valley to deposit sediments rich in the minerals chlorine, bromide, sulphate, bicarbonate, magnesium, sodium, calcium, iodine and potassium. Once filtered, cleansed and sterilized, the mud – with its glossy black appearance, velvet texture and slightly sulphurous smell – has many therapeutic benefits.

Dead Sea mineral salts and mud have a balancing effect on skin cells, normalizing cell turnover and encouraging the elimination of toxins. They are highly effective treatments for skin conditions such as eczema and psoriasis. During treatment, skin feels stimulated, taut and invigorated. Oils, dirt and sweat are lifted out of the pores, allowing the skin to feel glowing, soft, smooth and more elastic.

Raw mineral mud should not be used on the face. Opt instead for gentler, specially formulated mud masks that are designed for facial use.

Warm mineral mud-wrap treatments can help to reduce fluid retention by stimulating the circulation. They cause a light sweat, dilate blood vessels and have a natural diuretic effect on the kidneys. Excess fluid is also thought to be drawn out of the tissues by the osmotic effect of the mud.

Facials

A self-administered facial will leave you feeling cleansed, refreshed and relaxed, but there is nothing to beat a professional facial. This provides a skin analysis, steaming and deep cleansing of the pores to extract blackheads and whiteheads, massage, a mask or exfoliating peel, followed by remoisturizing. During detox, and provided your finances allow it, you could indulge in a facial once a week – trying different techniques and products – then enter a maintenance programme of facials on a monthly basis using the method you like best. A facial that includes lymphatic drainage massage is especially helpful during detox.

Hydrotherapy

The healing power of water is harnessed in the treatment known as hydrotherapy. It takes the form of bathing, but this could be in essential oils, spa waters, seaweed or algae extracts, mineral muds, herbs, peat and sea waters. Temperature plays an important role in hydrotherapy. Cold baths are refreshing and stimulating, while warm water is relaxing; hot water opens the pores and promotes the elimination of toxins through sweating. Hot baths should be avoided during detox because they open up blood vessels in the skin and can lead to feelings of faintness.

It's easy to indulge in hydrotherapy at home, but you might need to alter your bath or shower. A few simple changes, such as lighting the bathroom with candles, or scenting the air with sensual aromatherapy oils, can bring a new dimension to bathtime.

Try adding a 250-g (8-oz) sachet of Dead Sea mineral salts to a warm bath and lie back in the relaxing waters for 20 minutes. (**Note:** Avoid contact with the eyes, and cover cuts or grazes with Vaseline or they will sting).

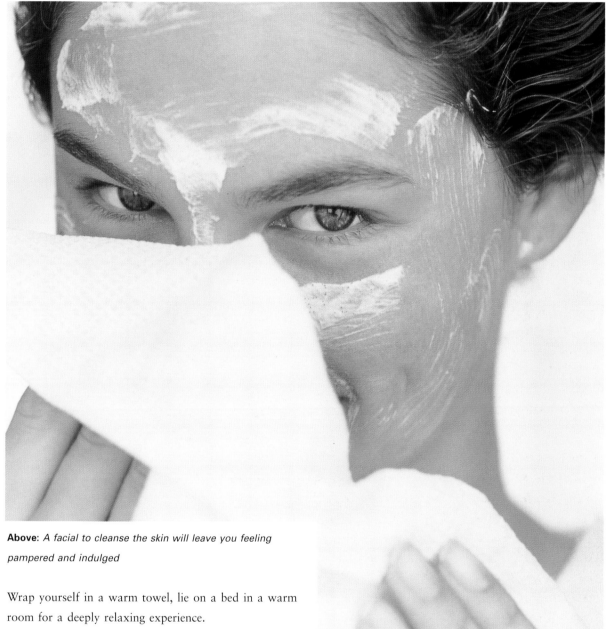

Above: *A facial to cleanse the skin will leave you feeling pampered and indulged*

Wrap yourself in a warm towel, lie on a bed in a warm room for a deeply relaxing experience.

Alternatively, add diluted neroli oil or other relaxing bath product to warm water and relax for 15 minutes. Keep several blends at home so that you can select one to suit any particular mood.

Saunas

A truly hot sauna is not advised during full-scale detox as it opens up all the blood vessels in the skin and can lead to dizziness. Saunas are best enjoyed at the end of a detox programme, once you are in the maintenance phase of eating a healthy diet and following a healthy lifestyle. Always drink plenty of water when sitting in a sauna.

Steam treatment

Steam treatments can be applied just to the face, or to the whole body. For best results, use a walk-in steam cabinet in a gym or salon, which is perfumed with relaxing aromatherapy oils. Many toxins are stored in the layer of fatty tissues just under the skin, and steam rooms help to mobilize and release them through the skin by promoting sweating. Sit in the warm cocoon, close your eyes and meditate, while imagining all the toxins oozing out of your pores and trickling away.

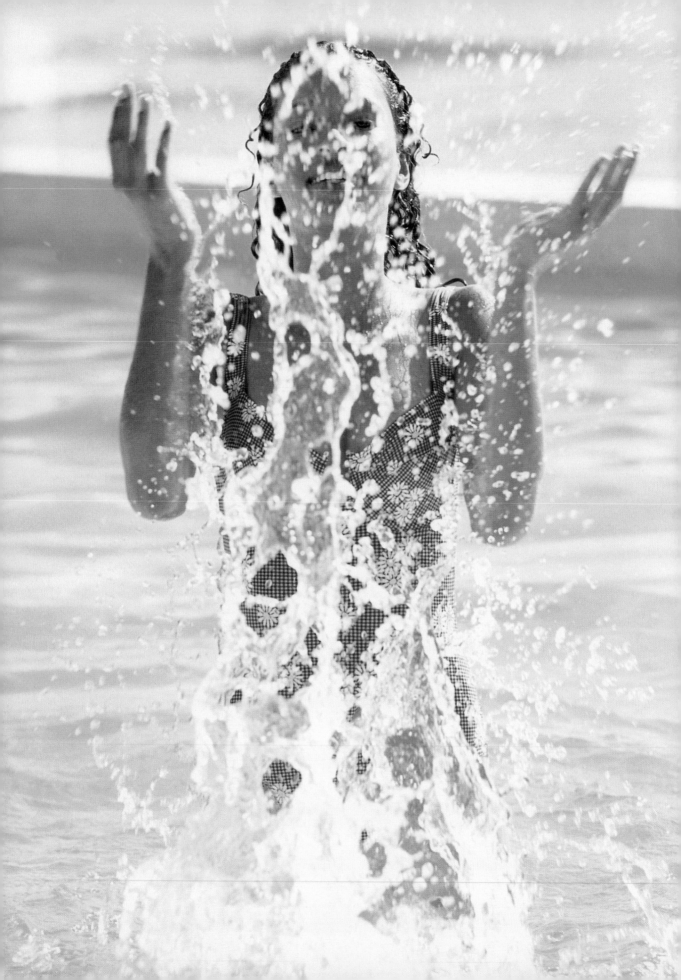

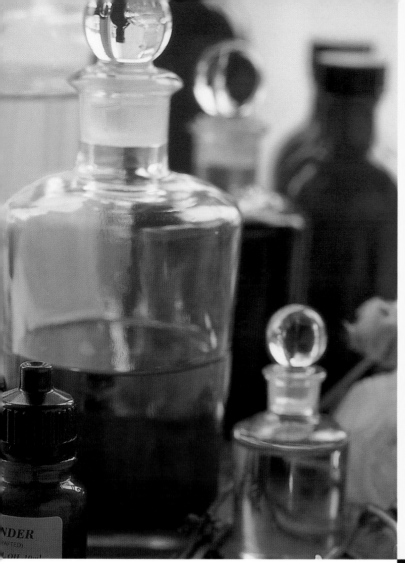

Enjoy life to the full

– build love, laughter

and fun into every

part of your life and

relationships for

total fulfilment and

an all-round sense

of wellbeing.

Enjoy

One of the side effects of a toxic lifestyle is loss of sex drive. This can result from a number of factors, of which stress, poor diet, lack of sleep, physical unfitness and over-indulgence in alcohol are major culprits. Certain medical conditions can also lead to loss of libido. These include pregnancy, menopause, hysterectomy, prostate problems and underactive testicles.

After following a detox programme, you might find that your libido improves. This can be helped by certain herbal supplements that have a natural aphrodisiac action, such as Chinese ginseng, gotu kola and pfaffia (see pages 63–66). If your sex drive needs an extra boost, however, the following essential oils and herbal remedies can help get your desire back on track.

AROMATHERAPY AS APHRODISIAC

Try combining three of the following aromatherapy oils to make your own sensual aphrodisiac blends.

ESSENTIAL OIL *	FOR LOW SEX DRIVE LINKED WITH PHYSICAL TIREDNESS OR MENTAL EXHAUSTION	FOR LOW SEX DRIVE LINKED WITH STRESS, OVERWORK OR INSOMNIA
Angelica	✳	
Benzoin	✳	✳
Bergamot		✳
Black pepper	✳	
Clary sage		✳
Coriander		✳
Fennel		✳
Geranium		✳
Grapefruit		✳
Jasmine		✳
Juniper berry		✳
Lavender		✳
Lemon	✳	
Neroli		✳
Orange	✳	✳
Patchouli		✳
Peppermint	✳	
Pine	✳	
Rose		✳
Rosemary	✳	
Rosewood	✳	✳
Sandalwood	✳	✳
Vanilla		✳
Vetiver		✳
Ylang-ylang		✳

The following combinations are popular, but the balance in which they are blended together depends on your personal taste.

✧ Black pepper and Ylang-ylang

✧ Benzoin, Rose and Vanilla

✧ Lavender, Geranium and Ylang-ylang

✧ Rose, Lemon and Vanilla

✧ Black pepper, Geranium, Sandalwood and Ylang-ylang

✧ Jasmine, Neroli and Orange

Below: *Rose petals contain sensual aromatic oils*

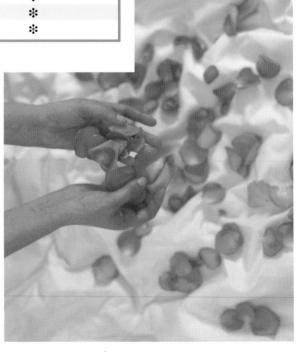

✳ Essential oils should always be diluted in a carrier oil, such as almond, jojoba or wheatgerm, before being massaged into the skin or added to bath water. Add a maximum total of two drops essential oil to each 5 ml (60 drops) of carrier oil.

When making up a blend, choose oils whose aromas you like, and preferably those that your partner likes, too. Experiment until you find an aroma that pleases you and best suits your mood. Keep a note of the total number of drops used so that you can ensure it is correctly diluted with carrier oil. Altogether, every five drops of essential oil should be balanced with 10 ml (120 drops) of carrier oil.

Prosexual herbal supplements

The herbal supplements with the most useful prosexual effects include catuaba, damiana, muira puama and tribulus.

Catuaba (Erythroxylon catuaba)

Extracts from the bark of catuaba – also known as the tree of love – are widely used in Central America to increase the sex drive, especially in older males. However, the plant's aromatic chemicals promote erotic dreams and increased sexual energy in both men and women. Erotic dreams usually start within 5–21 days of taking extracts regularly, and these are followed by increased sexual desire. Catuaba also improves peripheral blood flow and can improve erectile dysfunction.

Dose: 1g on waking and 1g on going to bed, capsule/tablet.

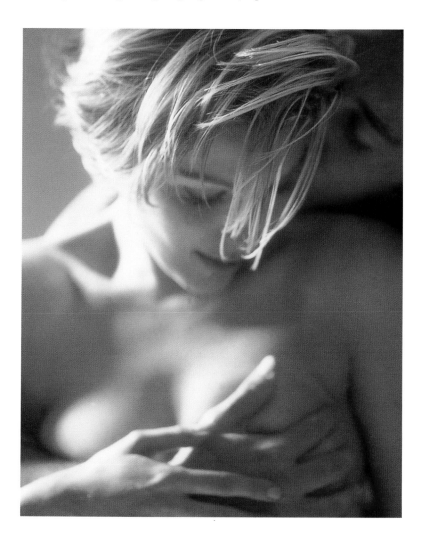

Damiana (Turnera diffusa aphrodisiaca)

A small shrub with aromatic leaves, which have been used as an aphrodisiac since the time of the Mayans. It contains aromatic oils that have a gentle stimulatory effect on the genitals to produce localized tingling and throbbing sensations. It is especially helpful where low sex drive is linked with anxiety or mild depression. It is usually taken on an occasional basis – when needed rather than regularly. Some evidence suggests that it might reduce iron absorption from the gut, so it should not be used long term.

Dose: 200–800 mg per day in capsule form.

Muira puama (Ptychopetalum olacoides)

Also known as potency wood, muira puama is a small tree found in the Brazilian rainforest. Its roots and bark are taken to enhance sexual desire and help overcome impotence, but researchers are unsure how it works. It is thought to stimulate sexual desire through a direct action on brain chemicals, through stimulating nerve endings in the genitals and by boosting the function of testosterone. Muira puama is also used as a general tonic for the nervous system.

Dose: 1–1.5 g capsule/tablet per day for 10–14 days.

Tribulus (Tribulus terrestris)

This Indian plant, also known as *ci ji li*, used in ayurvedic medicine. A five-day course has been shown to increase testosterone levels in some healthy men, and to improve the loss of sex drive linked with lethargy, fatigue and the so-called male menopause. Tribulus has diuretic actions and is traditionally used as a general male tonic and as a liver stimulant.

Dose: 250mg per day or one three times per day in capsules standardized to contain 40 per cent furostanol saponins.

Left: *Massaging diluted aromatherapy oils into the skin can transform your love life*

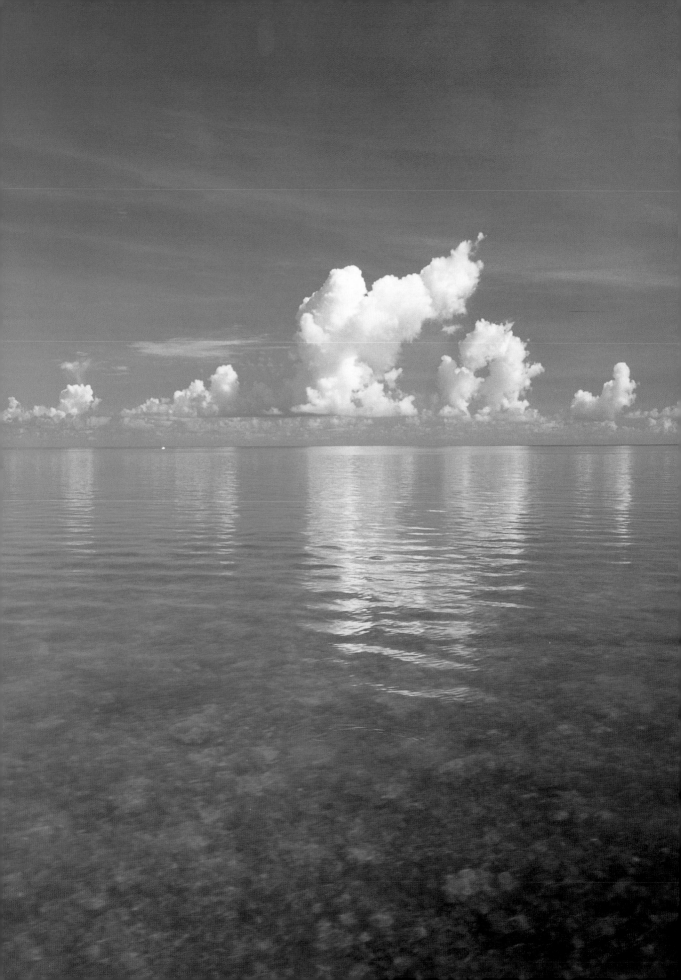

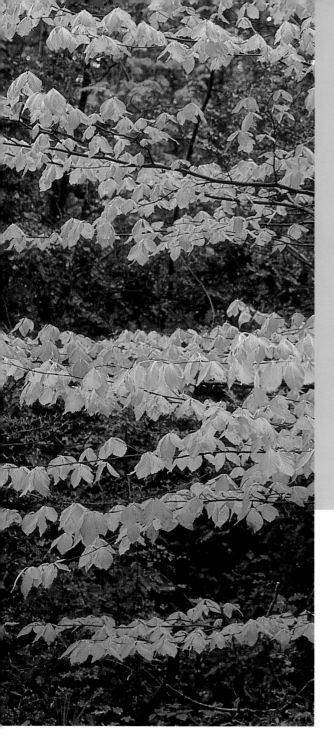

Feng shui is an ancient Chinese practice based on the belief that minimizing clutter and changing the position of certain items within the home can improve the flow of energy in a room.

CHAPTER TEN

Live

While detoxing your body, you might also find it useful to simplify your surroundings. Just looking at an untidy room heaped with discarded papers, books and other items can make you feel oppressed, while surrounding yourself with clean, clear surfaces can help you feel more relaxed and calm. Feng shui is an ancient Chinese practice based on the belief that minimizing clutter and changing the position of certain items within the home can improve the flow of energy in a room. Bringing some of the principles of feng shui into your home as part of your detox programme can have a therapeutic effect on many aspects of your life, including health, wealth and happiness. You can read up on it in one of the many books now available on the subject, or have your home assessed by a feng shui consultant for a professional make-over.

Feng Shui

Meaning "wind and water", feng shui is the Chinese art of arranging one's life in accordance with the forces of the universe. Its beliefs are based on three natural harmonies:

- the harmony that exists between an individual and the immediate environment
- the harmony that exists between the environment and its broader surroundings
- the larger harmony that exists among the energies converging on a particular person in any particular space

These energy patterns acting on your home are considered to be among the most important influences on relaxation, good health and prosperity. Even subtle changes, such as the placement of an eight-sided mirror near your front door, can have dramatic protective effects.

According to the rules of feng shui, creams, off-whites and beiges are suitable for any room, while light green is auspicious for bathrooms and sitting rooms, yellows and strong earth colours for the kitchen, and soft peach or pink tones for sleeping areas. Vibrant reds and oranges are considered overpowering and unsuitable for use in the home, while blue – especially dark blue – is believed to be inauspicious because it is the colour of water, which can absorb and store energy in an unpredictable and troubling way.

Below: *Light, colour and plants should form balance in your living space*

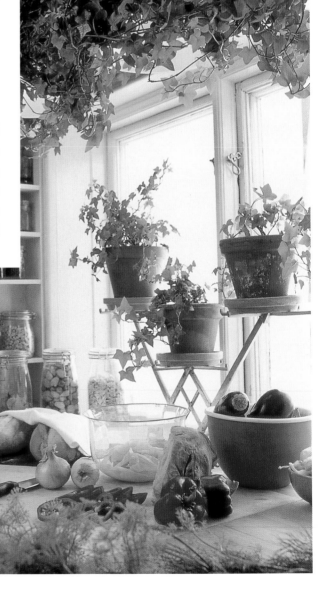

Sympathetic lighting is also important for it is beneficial effects on wellbeing. Allowing shimmering daylight to pass through lightweight muslin or voile curtains can transform the atmosphere of a room. At night-time a softer mood can be created by having several low-wattage lamps dotted around a room instead of one overhead light. Uplighters and dimmer-switches are especially effective at creating a feeling of restfulness.

Colour plays an important role in your home, too. Use the healing power of green plants for relaxation, and for restful effects use the Earth's palate of natural colours – muted greens, creams and beiges – with rich yet subtle shades of ochre or cinnamon. Natural textures, such as slate, wood, pebbles, linen, cotton and hessian, also contribute to a restful atmosphere.

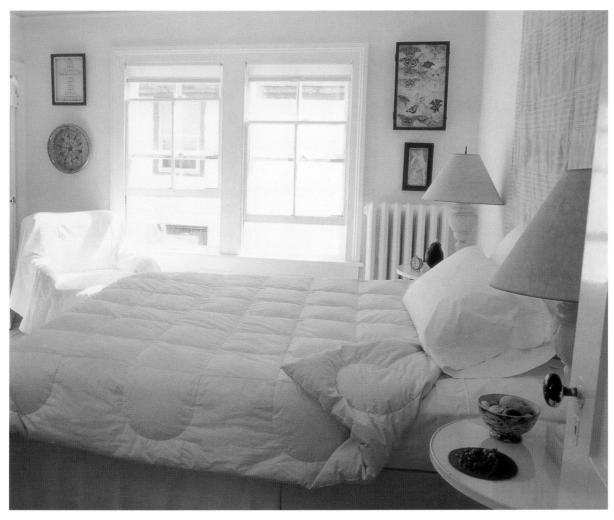

Above: *The way energy flows in your bedroom can affect the quality of sleep*

Tips to Detox Your Home

- Clear out all unnecessary clutter.
- Carefully consider which ornaments or pictures are really necessary.
- Go through drawers and cupboards one at a time, retaining only what is really necessary; things you are unsure of can be consigned to the loft.
- Clear all work surfaces at the end of each day. Place reminders about tasks still outstanding in a "To do" tray to ensure that you address them as soon as possible.
- Don't allow any clutter to accumulate under your bed.
- Throw away all out-of-date medicines.
- Use colour to freshen a room, taking care to use non-toxic paints.
- Consider giving away any clothes you haven't worn for at least a year.
- Define the purpose of each room and try not to fit too much into one space. If you must allow a bedroom to double as a home office, for example, separate the two areas with a screen.
- Use recordings of natural sounds, such as birdsong, waterfalls or ocean waves, to add a restful new dimension to your home (see Resources, page 126).
- Use aromatherapy to scent your room with a relaxing perfume.

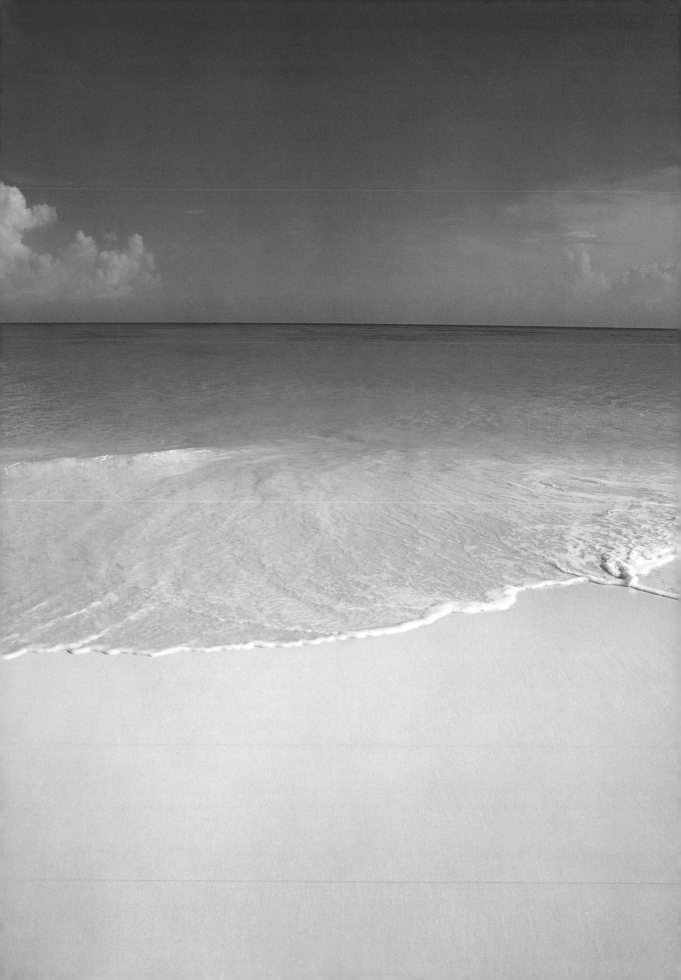

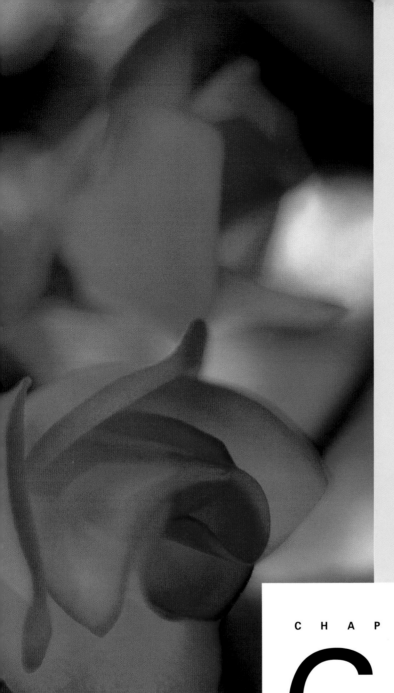

As well as detoxing your lifestyle and body, you need to purge harmful, negative – or toxic – thoughts from your mind and learn to love and look after yourself.

CHAPTER ELEVEN

Grow

Total detox needs to address the mind as well as the body to help you shed potentially harmful thought patterns and habits that can increase the chance of ill health. Psychologists have identified a number of faulty – or toxic – thought patterns that can lead to irrational fears and which need to be discarded. Try to avoid the following common mistakes.

Toxic thought patterns

Labels: "I'm a loser." "I'm stupid." "I'm not good enough."
Negative projections: "He must think I'm stupid." "They must be fed up with me now."
Negative predictions: "I know I'm going to fail." "He's bound to say no."

Negative generalizations: "I always get things wrong." "Everyone's against me."

Turning positives into negatives: "They only invited me to make up the numbers." "That lucky guess was a sheer fluke."

Thinking in black-and-white terms: "He's either with me or against me."

Raising the stakes: "This is the worst thing that's ever happened to me." "I can't stand this any more."

Accepting inappropriate blame: "My team lost – it's all my fault for not supporting them enough."

Blaming others: "It's all their fault – they should have seen this coming."

Belittling positives: "I've managed to stop smoking, but so what? I still drink too much."

Thinking emotionally: "She upset me – she must be a really unpleasant person." "I can't cope with that now; let's forget about it and it will go away."

Thinking in shoulds: "You should do this." "You should have said so." Instead, try saying, "I would appreciate it if you…"

Thinking in oughts: "I ought to say yes." "I ought to try harder." Instead, trying saying, "I would prefer to…"

Thinking in musts: "I must do this." "I must say yes." Instead, try saying, "I intend to…"

Thinking in have tos: "I have to do this." "I have to try harder." Instead, try saying, "I would like to…"

Using extremes: "My result was terrible." "I was dreadful." Instead, use milder terms, such as "annoying", "unfortunate" or "inconvenient".

One of the most effective ways to detox your thoughts is to turn destructive, negative thoughts into positive ones so that:

✧ "I can't cope" becomes "I *can* cope."
✧ "I can't do this" becomes "I *can* do this."
✧ "I'm useless" becomes "I *am* useful."
✧ "This is too difficult" becomes "I look forward to this challenge."

TIPS FOR PERSONAL GROWTH

• Realign your priorities and aim for things worth being rather than things worth having.

• Give up being an idealist or perfectionist.
• Accept that things can and will go wrong, and do not automatically look for someone to blame.
• Seek out positive points rather than excuses to be disappointed.
• Give praise where praise is due.
• Say thank you more often so that people know you appreciate their efforts.
• Listen to what others have to say.
• Learn to laugh at yourself rather than at other people.
• Be more patient.
• Take regular time out to relax during the day.
• Put aside one evening a week for personal pleasure.
• Talk about your emotions rather than bottling them up.

Bach flower remedies

These homoeopathic preparations are designed to help a variety of emotional states, including those associated with toxic thoughts. The remedies contain flower essences preserved in grape alcohol and are used to alleviate physical symptoms by treating underlying emotional problems.

Dr Bach classified emotional problems into seven major groups, further subdivided into a total of 38 negative or harmful states of mind. For each of these emotional states, a complementary flower essence can restore emotional balance.

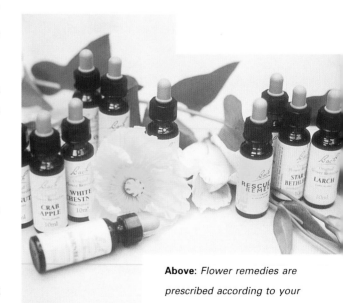

Above: *Flower remedies are prescribed according to your emotional traits*

The most well known of the Bach essences is Rescue Remedy – a combination of five flower essences (rock rose, impatiens, clematis, star of Bethlehem and cherry plum) that is used to help obtain emotional balance during times of crisis or stress. The full range of remedies and their uses are listed below.

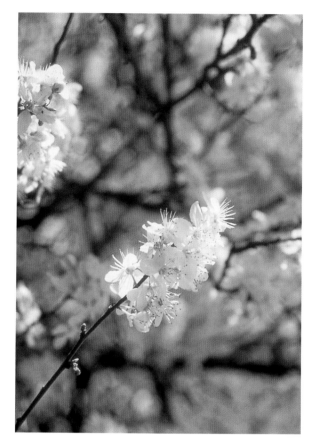

Above: *Flower essences such as cherry blossom are used to make emotionally balancing remedies*

The preparation and use of Bach flower remedies

There are two main ways in which Bach remedies are prepared. Both methods follow homoeopathic principles.

Infusion: Flowerheads are placed on the surface of a small glass bowl filled with pure spring water. This is left to infuse in direct sunlight for three hours, then the flowers are discarded and the infused spring water preserved in grape alcohol. This resulting solution is called the mother tincture, which is further diluted to create the individual stock remedies.

Boiling: Short lengths of flower-bearing twigs are boiled in pure spring water for 30 minutes. The plant material is then discarded and the water allowed to cool, before being preserved in grape alcohol. The resulting solution is the mother tincture, which will be further diluted for use.

To use: Place two drops of a flower remedy straight on to your tongue, or put two drops in a glass of water and sip the liquid until the symptoms have passed. If necessary, up to seven remedies can be mixed together at a time.

To blend: Place two drops of up to seven selected remedies in a 30 ml dropper bottle and top up with plain mineral water. Take four drops of this individually tailored mix four times a day, or more frequently if needed.

Ailments and Their Bach Remedies
Fear

✧ Rock rose (*Helianthemum nummularium*) for extreme terror, panic, fright and nightmares.

✧ Mimulus (*Mimulus guttatus*) for known fears and phobias, timidity and shyness.

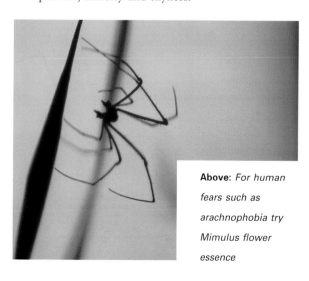

Above: *For human fears such as arachnophobia try Mimulus flower essence*

⬥ Cherry plum (*Prunus cerasifera*) for fear of losing control, uncontrollable rages, tempers, impulses, fear of causing harm to oneself or others.

⬥ Aspen (*Populus tremula*) for vague fears and anxieties of unknown origin, sense of foreboding, apprehension or impending doom.

⬥ Red chestnut (*Aesculus carnea*) for excessive fear or over-concern for others.

Uncertainty and indecision

⬥ Cerato (*Ceratostigma willmottianum*) for those who doubt their own ability to judge situations or make decisions.

⬥ Scleranthus (*Scleranthus annus*) for the indecisive and those subject to swings in energy or mood.

⬥ Gentian (*Gentianella amarella*) for the easily discouraged, those who hesitate, are despondent or self-doubting.

⬥ Gorse (*Ulex europaeus*) (pictured below) for feelings of despair, hopelessness and futility.

⬥ Hornbeam (*Carpinus betulus*) for "Monday morning" feelings of not being able to face the day, tiredness, procrastination, and those needing inner strength.

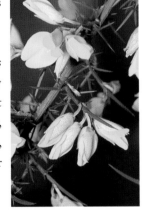

⬥ Wild oat (*Bromus ramosus*) for those dissatisfied with their current lifestyle or career, and who cannot decide which alternative path to follow.

Insufficient interest in present circumstances

⬥ Clematis (*Clematis vitalba*) for escapists, who live more in the future than the present, lack of concentration, daydreaming, lack of interest in present circumstances, out-of-body sensations.

⬥ Honeysuckle (*Lonicera caprifolium*) for those living too much in the past, nostalgia, homesickness.

⬥ Wild rose (*Rosa canina*) for apathy, resignation to circumstances, making little effort to improve situations or find happiness.

⬥ Olive (*Olea europaea*) for total exhaustion, mental or physical weariness, sapped vitality, especially during convalescence.

⬥ White chestnut (*Aesculus hippocastanum*) for persistent, unwanted thoughts, mental arguments, preoccupation with worry

⬥ Mustard (*Sinapis arvensis*) for deep gloom descending for no apparent reason, melancholy and heavy sadness.

⬥ Chestnut bud (*Aesculus hippocastanum*) for those who fail to learn from their mistakes.

Loneliness

⬥ Water violet (*Hottonia palustris*) for those who prefer to be alone, or are superior, aloof, proud and reserved in attitude; for those who will advise but do not get personally involved in others' problems.

⬥ Impatiens (*Impatiens glandulifera*) for those who are quick in thought and action but irritable or impatient, especially with those who are slower.

⬥ Heather (*Calluna vulgaris*) for excessive talkativeness and those constantly seeking companionship and an ear to listen; for the self-absorbed, who find difficulty in being alone.

Over-sensitivity to influences and ideas

⬥ Agrimony (*Agrimonia eupatoria*) for those not wishing to burden others, covering problems up with a cheerful façade, for those seeking out company and good times to avoid facing up to their problems.

✧ Centaury (*Centaurium umbellatum*) for those who cannot say no, for the subservient, those who are anxious to please and easily exploited.

✧ Walnut (*Juglans regia*) for stabilizing the emotions during periods of transition, such as puberty and the menopause; for adjusting to new beginnings or relationships.

✧ Holly (*Ilex aquifolium*) for negative feelings, such as envy, suspicion, revenge or hatred.

Despondency or despair

✧ Larch (*Larix decidua*) for those lacking in self-confidence, who anticipate failure and make little effort to succeed.

✧ Pine (*Pinus sylvestris*) for self-reproach, guilt and those who are not satisfied with their own actions; for those who blame themselves for the misfortunes of others.

✧ Elm (*Ulmus procera*) for those who overextend themselves, are overwhelmed or burdened with responsibilities.

✧ Sweet chestnut (*Castanea sativa*) for those who have reached the limits of their endurance, for deep despair or unbearable anguish.

✧ Star of Bethlehem (*Ornithogalum umbellatum*) for mental and emotional stress following traumatic experiences or grief.

✧ Willow (*Salix vitellina*) for those who feel they have suffered unjust misfortune, and for resentfulness and bitterness.

✧ Oak (*Quercus robur*) for the brave and determined, who never usually give up, despite adversity or illness, but who are losing their strength to fight.

✧ Crab apple (*Malus pumila*) for feelings of shame, unworthiness, uncleanliness, poor self-image or fear of contamination; helps to detoxify and cleanse.

Over-control

✧ Chicory (*Cichorium intybus*) (pictured below) for those who like to keep their family and friends close by, and find it difficult to allow them to go their own way; for people who expect dutiful obedience in return for the love they give.

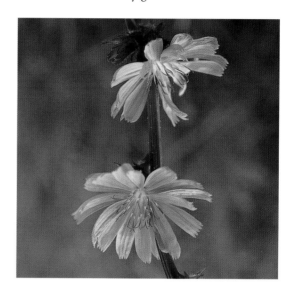

✧ Vervain (*Verbena officinalis*) for those with strong opinions, those incensed by injustice, the over-enthusiastic or argumentative.

✧ Vine (*Vitis vinifera*) for the strong-willed with a tendency to be ruthless, domineering, dictatorial or inflexible.

✧ Beech (*Fagus sylvatica*) for the critical and intolerant, those who seek perfection and are continually finding fault.

✧ Rock water (*Aqua petra*) for those who are overly strict with themselves, hard taskmasters with a severely disciplined lifestyle.

Select the most appropriate remedies for your needs and keep them with you at all times to use as necessary as part of your detox programme.

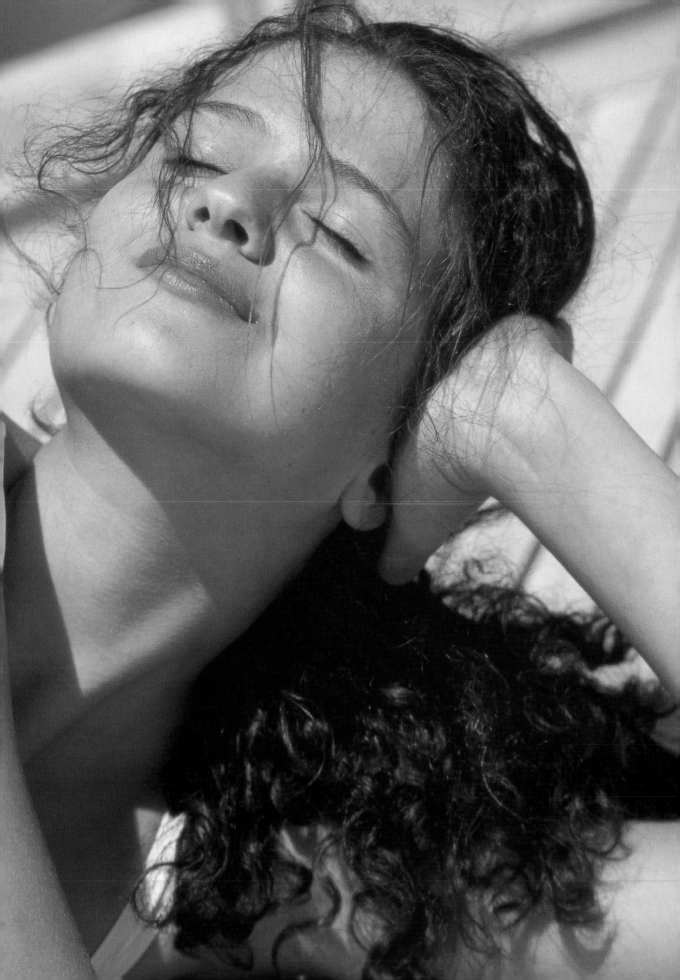

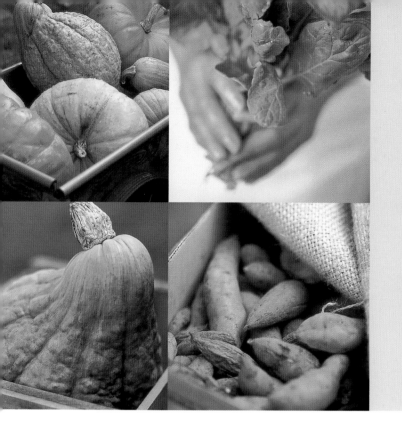

It is important to drink plenty of mineral or filtered (non-chlorinated) water to help flush toxins through your system. Aim to drink 3 litres (5 pints) of fluid per day.

total Detox plan

The logical progression for a cleansing and balancing detox diet is as follows:

✧ Start cleansing, dietary and lifestyle changes as the foundation of your detox plan.

✧ Take cleansing supplements to boost the body's eliminatory systems.

✧ Once cleansing is under way, add balancing nutritional supplements to support future health and immunity.

✧ Use complementary therapies to assist the detox process.

The rationale for this sequence is that there is little point in adding nutritional supplements to a system that is already toxic: that would be like adding clean oil to dirty oil when servicing a car – a complete waste of time and effort.

During the cleansing process, you can, if you wish, help to increase the elimination of toxins by raising a sweat with exercise or steam rooms. Go easy with saunas, as excess heat during detox can cause fainting. If you do decide to indulge in a sauna, make sure you are accompanied by a companion, and drink plenty of fluids. Ideally, saunas should wait until you are back to eating a normal yet healthy diet. Alternatively, you could take a sauna the day before you start the full detox programme to get you off to a good start. Supplements that promote sweating and urinary flow, such as dandelion, can also be used if you wish.

It is important to drink plenty of mineral or filtered (non-chlorinated) water to help flush toxins through your system. Aim to drink 3 litres (5 pints) of fluid per day. For variety you might like to include fruit and herbal teas, which can be drunk throughout the cleansing diet.

Following a cleansing and balancing diet has the useful side effect of promoting healthy bowel function because it increases fibre intake and replenishes levels of friendly bacteria (e.g. *Lactobacillus acidophilus*). Make sure you have only fruit, juices, vegetables, rice and so forth that has been certified organic.

Some people like to fast at the beginning of detox, using just water or juices. This should ideally be done under the supervision of a qualified practitioner as the liberation of excess toxins in the body can make you feel nauseated (see page 23).

Cutting out caffeine

During detox, you must cut caffeine out altogether. If you have previously had a high intake, however, you might suffer withdrawal symptoms, with headache and irritability. If you drink more than three caffeinated drinks per day, it is worth preparing yourself for detox by cutting down gradually on caffeine for a week or two before starting the cleansing diet.

Aluminium cookware

Replace all aluminium cookware with stainless steel equivalents.
Aluminium may be leached out into food during cooking – especially when preparing acidic dishes – and may build up in the body to produce toxic effects.

The total detox plan

The following detox plan will guide you through a simple cleansing and balancing diet that you can follow for 10 days. Do check that it is safe for you to follow this plan (see Chapter 1, page 11) and be sure to fill in the assessment plan on page 15 before you start.

During the cleansing phase of the programme, consume only:
- organic fresh fruit, vegetables and juices
- cooked brown rice
- organic wholemeal cereals
- live bio yoghurt
- plain cottage cheese
- pure mineral or spring water

You may eat as much or as little as you wish, but aim to eat at least half your normal daily energy intake to protect the lean tissues in your body (see page 24).

Eat little and often throughout the day. A typical intake of brown rice (uncooked weight) would be 50 g (2 oz) eaten 2–4 times throughout the day – a maximum daily intake of 225g (8 oz).

In addition, you might wish to make up a thin soup using fresh organic vegetables, herbs and black pepper (no salt) and eat this regularly throughout the day.

Fruit or vegetables juice may be diluted with spring water if you wish.

Some recipes require products to be soaked or marinated overnight, so check the next day's recipes for any preparation that must be made in advance. You do not need to stick to these plans or recipes at all strictly. If you prefer to eat just rice, soups, steamed vegetables and fruit, that is absolutely fine.

Cleansing Vegetable Soup (Serves 4)

4 garlic cloves
4 large tomatoes
1 kg (2 ¼ lb) mixed organic vegetables, e.g. onion, leek, potato, swede, parsnip, white cabbage, courgette, chard, beetroot, peppers, watercress, broccoli, celery, carrots, spinach, celeriac, fennel
bouquet garni (optional)
freshly ground black pepper
2 tablespoons chopped fresh herbs
freshly squeezed juice of 1 lemon

Clean and chop all the ingredients and place in a large pan with the bouquet garni, if using. Cover with water and boil until the vegetables are just soft.

Season with black pepper and add the fresh herbs and lemon juice.

The soup may be puréed if you wish, and frozen in individual portions to use throughout your detox.

Cleansing: day 1

On waking: Warm water flavoured with freshly squeezed lemon juice.

Breakfast: Fruit juice of your choice; prunes or figs soaked overnight in fruit juice or herbal tea; live bio yoghurt.

Mid-morning: Banana and other easily digested fruits such as oranges, apples, pears and melons, as often as you wish.

Lunch: Cooked brown rice, cottage cheese, large mixed salad with crudités (e.g. carrot, celery, courgette) and a sprinkling of nuts and seeds; live bio yoghurt; carrot and/or apple juice.

Mid-afternoon: Mixed fruit and vegetable crudités, as often as you wish.

Dinner: Cooked brown rice, large bowl of vegetable soup (see page 114); live bio yoghurt.

Evening: Fresh fruit as often as you wish.

Drink at least 3 litres (5 pints) of mineral water, fruit juice or herbal teas per day.

Suggested cleansing supplements

Psyllium husks (1–2 tablespoons at night before going to bed)

Standardized milk thistle extracts

Dandelion root extracts

Humic acids

If prone to constipation, try aloe vera

Antioxidants

Vitamin C (1 g, preferably as Ester-C, three times per day)

Vitamin E (286 mg per day)

Selenium (200 mcg daily)

Choose your own

Exercise of the day...

Complementary therapy of the day ....

Relaxation of the day ....

Indulgence of the day...

Go to bed early – no later than 9 p.m. – to rest and rejuvenate.

Adding crunch and flavour

Sprinkle any of the following on to salads, rice or main meals whenever you like.

50g (2 oz) sunflower seeds, toasted and/or raw

50g (2 oz) pumpkin seeds, toasted and/or raw

100g (4oz) mixed unsalted nuts

50g (2 oz) pine kernels

50g (2 oz) sesame seeds, toasted

50g (2 oz) poppy seeds

Cleansing: day 2

On waking: Warm water flavoured with freshly squeezed lemon juice.

Breakfast: Fruit juice of your choice; prunes or figs soaked overnight in water or herbal tea; live bio yoghurt.

Mid-morning: Banana and other easily digested fruits, such as oranges, apples, pears and melons, as often as you wish.

Lunch: Brown rice salad; cottage cheese with avocado; grated raw beetroot, carrot and courgette; large mixed salad with a sprinkling of nuts and seeds; live bio yoghurt; carrot and/or apple juice.

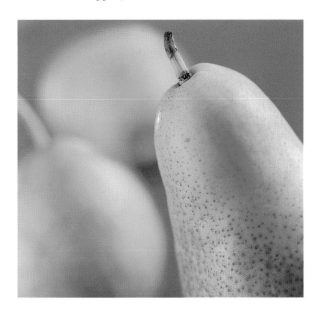

Mid-afternoon: Mixed fruit and vegetable crudités, as often as you wish.

Dinner: Cooked brown rice, large bowl of vegetable soup (see page 114); live bio yoghurt.

Evening: Fresh fruit as often as you wish.

Drink at least 3 litres (5 pints) of mineral water, fruit juice or herbal teas per day.

Suggested cleansing supplements

Psyllium husks (1–2 tablespoons at night before going to bed)

Standardized milk thistle extracts

Dandelion root extracts

Humic acids

If prone to constipation, try aloe vera

Antioxidants

Vitamin C (1 g, preferably as Ester-C, three times per day)

Vitamin E (286 mg per day)

Selenium (200 mcg daily)

Choose your own

Exercise of the day..

Complementary therapy of the day ....

Relaxation of the day ....

Indulgence of the day..

Go to bed early – no later than 9 p.m. – to rest and rejuvenate.

Detox Fennel Soup (Serves 4)

- 450 g (1 lb) Florence fennel bulbs, thinly sliced
- 1 large onion, chopped
- 3 garlic cloves, crushed
- 3 beef tomatoes, sliced
- 1 tablespoon chopped fresh parsley
- 1 tablespoon chopped fresh basil
- 1 glass tomato or vegetable juice
- freshly ground black pepper
- chopped nuts and seeds, for garnish

Place all the ingredients (except the seasoning) in a saucepan and top up with enough water to cover vegetables. Cover and simmer gently for 30 minutes.

Season with black pepper and sprinkle with a few chopped nuts and seeds before serving.

This soup can be frozen in individual portions, if you wish, to use throughout your detox.

Cleansing: day 3

On waking: Warm water flavoured with freshly squeezed lemon juice.

Breakfast: Fruit juice of your choice; prunes or figs soaked overnight in water or herbal tea; live bio yoghurt.

Mid-morning: Banana and other easily digested fruits, such as oranges, apples, pears and melons, as often as you wish.

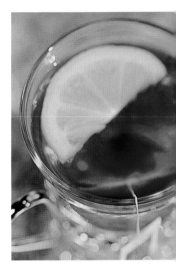

Lunch: Brown rice salad; hummus; crudités; Greek salad; live bio yoghurt; carrot and/or apple juice.

Mid-afternoon: Mixed fruit and vegetable crudités, as often as you wish.

Dinner: Cooked brown rice, large bowl of ratatouille (see page 117); live bio yoghurt.

Evening: Fresh fruit as often as you wish.

Drink at least 3 litres (5 pints) of mineral water, fruit juice or herbal teas per day.

Suggested cleansing supplements

Psyllium husks (1–2 tablespoons at night before going to bed)

Standardized milk thistle extracts

Dandelion root extracts

Humic acids

If prone to constipation, try aloe vera

Antioxidants

Vitamin C (1 g, preferably as Ester-C, three times per day)

Vitamin E (286 mg per day)

Selenium (200 mcg daily)

Choose your own

Exercise of the day...

Complementary therapy of the day ....

Relaxation of the day ....

Indulgence of the day...

Go to bed early – no later than 9 p.m. – to rest and rejuvenate.

Detox Ratatouille (Serves 4)

- 1 large onion, sliced
- 2 garlic cloves, crushed
- Small piece root ginger, peeled and finely chopped
- 1 large sweet red pepper, deseeded and sliced lengthways
- 1 large aubergine, chopped
- 1 large courgette, chopped
- 4 beefsteak tomatoes, chopped
- 1 tablespoon chopped fresh parsley
- 1 tablespoon chopped fresh basil
- 1 tablespoon chopped fresh coriander
- 1 teaspoon chopped fresh thyme
- freshly ground black pepper

Place all the ingredients (except the seasoning) in a saucepan, add enough water or tomato/vegetable juice to cover, and simmer with the lid on for 30 minutes. Stir occasionally. Season to taste with black pepper. This soup can be frozen in individual portions, if you wish, to use throughout your detox.

Detox Hummus (Serves 4)

- 150g (5 oz) dried chickpeas, soaked overnight until their weight has more or less doubled
- 3 tablespoons extra virgin olive oil
- zest and freshly squeezed juice of 2 lemons
- 3 garlic cloves, crushed
- 120g (4 ½ oz) organic tahini (sesame) paste
- freshly ground black pepper
- chopped fresh parsley or ground paprika, for garnish

Drain the soaked chickpeas and transfer to a saucepan. Cover with fresh water and simmer for 1 ½ hours, or until soft. Drain, saving the liquid. Put

5 tablespoons of the cooking liquid in a blender with the olive oil, lemon zest, lemon juice and garlic. Start to blend, then slowly add the chickpeas and tahini paste. If the blender clogs, add more cooking liquid until a grainy purée is obtained. More olive oil or tahini paste can be added to vary the flavour as desired. Season to taste and garnish before serving.

Greek Salad (Serves 4)

- 225g (8 oz) mixed green salad leaves
- 8 whole radishes, trimmed
- 12 black olives, rinsed and stoned
- 12 green olives, rinsed and stoned
- 1 red onion, thinly sliced and separated into rings
- 1 red pepper, de-seeded and cut into strips
- 1 green pepper, de-seeded and cut into strips
- 1/4 cucumber, thinly sliced
- 8–12 cherry tomatoes
- 225g (8 oz) feta cheese
- coriander, for garnish

Arrange all the ingredients in a serving dish and garnish with the coriander.

Cleansing: day 4

On waking: Warm water flavoured with freshly squeezed lemon juice.

Breakfast: Fruit juice of your choice; prunes or figs soaked overnight in water or herbal tea; live bio yoghurt.

Mid-morning: Banana and other easily digested fruits, such as oranges, apples, pears and melons, as often as you wish.

Lunch: Cooked brown rice; cottage cheese and pineapple; grated raw beetroot, carrot and courgette; large mixed salad with a sprinkling of nuts and seeds; live bio yoghurt; carrot and/or apple juice.

Mid-afternoon: Mixed fruit and vegetable crudités, as often as you wish.

Dinner: Cooked brown rice; baked red peppers (see page 118); steamed broccoli; live bio yoghurt.

Evening: Fresh fruit as often as you wish.

Drink at least 3 litres (5 pints) of mineral water, fruit juice or herbal teas per day.

Suggested cleansing supplements

Psyllium husks (1–2 tablespoons at night before going to bed)

Standardized milk thistle extracts

Dandelion root extracts

Humic acids

If prone to constipation, try aloe vera

Antioxidants

Vitamin C (1 g, preferably as Ester-C, three times per day)

Vitamin E (286 mg per day)

Selenium (200 mcg daily)

Choose your own

Exercise of the day...

Complementary therapy of the day ....

Relaxation of the day ....

Indulgence of the day...

Go to bed early – no later than 9 p.m. – to rest and rejuvenate.

Detox Roasted Red Peppers (Serves 4)

- 4 large red peppers
- extra virgin olive oil
- 2 garlic cloves, crushed
- 2 tablespoons chopped fresh coriander
- 2 tablespoons chopped fresh basil
- freshly ground black pepper
- 4 beefsteak tomatoes, chopped
- 1 red chilli pepper, finely chopped
- cayenne pepper
- freshly squeezed juice of 1 lemon

Preheat the oven to 180ºC/350ºF/Gas Mark 4. Cut the red peppers in half through the stalk and remove the seeds. Lightly brush each pepper inside and out with the olive oil. Place the peppers on a baking sheet and distribute the garlic plus half the coriander and half the basil between them. Sprinkle with lemon juice and season with black pepper. Place some chopped tomato in each pepper half, then sprinkle with the chopped chilli and with cayenne pepper. Place the sheet in the oven and roast the peppers for 45–50 minutes, until the skins start to char. Garnish with the remaining basil and coriander leaves.

Cleansing: day 5

On waking: Warm water flavoured with freshly squeezed lemon juice.

Breakfast: Fruit juice of your choice; prunes or figs soaked overnight in water or herbal tea; live bio yoghurt.

Mid-morning: Banana and other easily digested fruits, such as oranges, apples, pears and melons, as often as you wish.

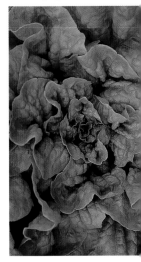

Lunch: Cooked brown rice; cottage cheese; warm green lentil, ginger and coriander salad; large mixed salad with a sprinkling of nuts and seeds; live bio yoghurt; carrot and/or apple juice.

Mid-afternoon: Mixed fruit and vegetable crudités, as often as you wish.

Dinner: Cooked brown rice; vegetable soup (see page 114); steamed broccoli; live bio yoghurt.

Evening: Fresh fruit as often as you wish.

Drink at least 3 litres (5 pints) of mineral water, fruit juice or herbal teas per day.

Suggested cleansing supplements

Psyllium husks (1–2 tablespoons at night before going to bed)

Standardized milk thistle extracts

Dandelion root extracts

Humic acids

If prone to constipation, try aloe vera

Antioxidants

Vitamin C (1 g, preferably as Ester-C, three times per day)

Vitamin E (286 mg per day)

Selenium (200 mcg daily)

Choose your own

Exercise of the day...

Complementary therapy of the day ....

Relaxation of the day ....

Indulgence of the day..

Go to bed early – no later than 9 p.m. – to rest and rejuvenate.

Green Lentil, Ginger and Coriander Salad

(Serves 4)

- 225g (8 oz) green lentils
- 600 ml (1 pint) water
- 1 large carrot, grated
- 1 tablespoon extra virgin olive oil
- 1 medium onion, finely chopped
- 2 garlic cloves, crushed
- 1 tablespoon coriander seed, crushed
- 2 tablespoons freshly squeezed lemon or lime juice
- 2.5-cm (1-in) piece root ginger, peeled and finely chopped
- freshly ground black pepper
- 1–2 tablespoons chopped fresh coriander, for garnish

Simmer the lentils in water for around 30 minutes, until they are cooked, but still firm. Add the grated carrot,cook for a further five minutes, then drain and set aside. Heat the olive oil and fry the onion, garlic and crushed coriander until beginning to colour. Add to the drained lentils with all the remaining ingredients, mix well and season with black pepper. Serve warm or cold, garnished with coriander leaves.

Balancing: day 6

On waking: Warm water flavoured with freshly squeezed lemon juice.

Breakfast: Fruit juice of your choice; mixed nuts, seeds and dried fruit muesli topped with semi-skimmed milk and live bio yoghurt.

Mid-morning: Banana and other easily digested fruits, such as oranges, apples, pears and melons, as often as you wish.

Lunch: Cooked brown rice; salade niçoise; live bio yoghurt; carrot and/or apple juice.

Mid-afternoon: Mixed fruit and vegetable crudités, as often as you wish.

Dinner: Cooked brown rice; grilled or steamed chicken breast; steamed carrots and broccoli; live bio yoghurt.

Evening: Fresh fruit as often as you wish.

Drink at least 3 litres (5 pints) of mineral water, fruit juice or herbal teas per day.

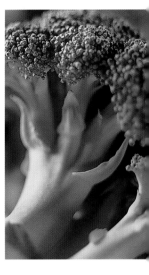

Suggested cleansing supplements

Psyllium husks (1–2 tablespoons at night before going to bed)

Standardized milk thistle extracts

Blue-green algae

If prone to constipation, try aloe vera

Antioxidants

Vitamin C (1 g, preferably as Ester-C, three times per day)

Vitamin E (286 mg per day)

Selenium (200 mcg daily)

Suggested balancing supplements

A vitamin and mineral supplement providing around 100 per cent of the recommended daily amount of as many micronutrients as possible

Evening primrose oil

An adaptogen, such as Siberian ginseng

Choose your own

Exercise of the day...

Complementary therapy of the day ....

Relaxation of the day ....

Indulgence of the day..

Detox Muesli (Makes 750 g/1 ½ lb)

Use organic ingredients.

- 50 g (2 oz) rolled oats
- 50 g (2 oz) toasted wheatflakes
- 50 g (2 oz) rye flakes

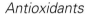

- 50 g (2 oz) barley flakes
- 50 g (2 oz) bran buds/flakes
- 100 g (4 oz) dried apricots, chopped
- 50 g (2 oz) dried dates, chopped
- 50 g (2 oz) dried figs, chopped
- 50 g (2 oz) walnuts, chopped
- 25 g (1 oz) Brazil nuts, chopped
- 25 g (1 oz) hazelnuts, chopped
- 50 g (2 oz) pine nuts
- 25 g (1 oz) sunflower seeds
- 25 g (1 oz) pumpkin seeds
- 25 g (1 oz) sesame seeds
- 25 g (1 oz) poppy seeds

Mix together all the ingredients, then store in an airtight container. Shake well before weighing out each serving, as the bran and small seeds tend to settle at the bottom

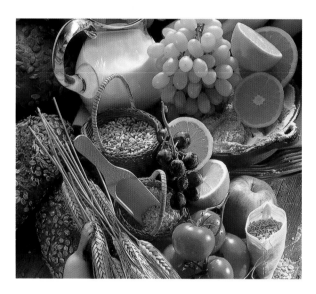

Salad Niçoise (Serves 4)

- 450 g (1 lb) French beans, topped and tailed
- 2 little gem lettuce hearts
- 8 small, new potatoes, boiled, cooled and halved
- 200 g (7 oz) fresh grilled tuna, cooled and flaked
- 2 hardboiled free-range eggs, shelled and chopped
- 12 black olives, stoned and halved
- 1 small onion, thinly sliced and separated into rings
- 12 cherry tomatoes

- extra virgin olive oil
- lime juice
- chopped fresh mint, chives and parsley

Cut the French beans in half lengthways and steam for 5–10 minutes, until tender but still crisp. Drain and plunge into icy cold water. Line a salad bowl with lettuce leaves. Arrange the potatoes and beans on top. Pile the flaked tuna fish into the middle of the bowl. Decorate round the edges with chopped egg, black olives and tomatoes. Drizzle with the olive oil and lime juice.

Balancing: day 7

On waking: Warm water flavoured with freshly squeezed lemon juice.

Breakfast: Fruit juice of your choice; mixed nuts, seeds and dried fruit muesli topped with semi-skimmed milk and live bio yoghurt.

Mid-morning: Banana and other easily digested fruits, such as oranges, apples, pears and melons, as often as you wish.

Lunch: Cooked brown rice; balancing bean salad; cottage cheese with pineapple; large mixed salad; live bio yoghurt; carrot and/or apple juice.

Mid-afternoon: Mixed fruit and vegetable crudités, as often as you wish.

Dinner: Boiled potatoes; grilled salmon steak; steamed broccoli; sweetcorn; live bio yoghurt.

Evening: Fresh fruit as often as you wish.

Drink at least 3 litres (5 pints) of mineral water, fruit juice or herbal teas per day.

Suggested cleansing supplements

Psyllium husks (1–2 tablespoons at night before going to bed)
Standardized milk thistle extracts
Blue-green algae
If prone to constipation, try aloe vera

Antioxidants

Vitamin C (1 g, preferably as Ester-C, three times per day)
Vitamin E (286 mg per day)
Selenium (200 mcg daily)

Suggested balancing supplements

A vitamin and mineral supplement providing around 100 per cent of the recommended daily amount of as many micronutrients as possible

Evening primrose oil

An adaptogen, such as Siberian ginseng

Choose your own

Exercise of the day...

Complementary therapy of the day ....

Relaxation of the day ....

Indulgence of the day..

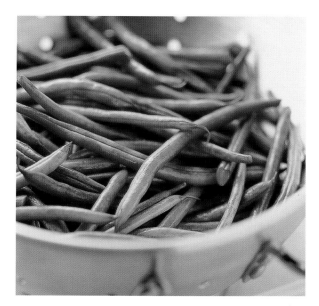

Balancing Bean Salad (Serves 4)

- 400 g (14 oz) mixed beans, cooked and cooled
- 1 beefsteak tomato, chopped
- 2 garlic cloves, crushed
- 2 tablespoons chopped fresh coriander
- few coriander seeds, crushed
- small piece root ginger, peeled and finely chopped
- 2 tablespoons chopped fresh parsley
- 2 tablespoons freshly squeezed lemon or lime juice
- 2 tablespoons freshly squeezed orange juice
- 4 tablespoons live bio yoghurt
- freshly ground black pepper

Mix all the ingredients together, season well and serve.

Grilled Salmon Steaks with Lemon and Herbs

(Serves 4)

- 1 tablespoon extra virgin olive oil
- 4 tablespoons freshly squeezed lemon or lime juice
- 2 spring onions, finely chopped
- 2 garlic cloves, crushed
- 4 tablespoons chopped fresh herbs (e.g. parsley, dill, rosemary, thyme)
- 4 x 100 g (4 oz) salmon steaks
- freshly ground black pepper

Mix together the olive oil, lemon juice, spring onions, garlic and fresh herbs. Marinate the salmon fillets in this mixture for at least 1 hour. Season well with black pepper, then cook under a hot grill until the salmon flesh is just set – about 4 minutes on each side. Baste with any leftover marinade during the cooking time.

Balancing: day 8

On waking: Warm water flavoured with freshly squeezed lemon juice.

Breakfast: Fruit juice of your choice; mixed nuts, seeds and dried fruit muesli topped with semi-skimmed milk and live bio yoghurt.

Mid-morning: Banana and other easily digested fruits, such as oranges, apples, pears and melons, as often as you wish.

Lunch: Mushroom, garlic and fennel soup (see page 122); large mixed salad; rice and mixed vegetable salad; live bio yoghurt; carrot and/or apple juice.

Mid-afternoon: Mixed fruit and vegetable crudités, as often as you wish.

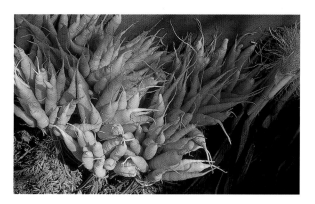

Dinner: Couscous; spicy chicken with lemon (this page); steamed broccoli and carrots; live bio yoghurt.

Evening: Fresh fruit as often as you wish.

Drink at least 3 litres (5 pints) of mineral water, fruit juice or herbal teas per day.

Suggested cleansing supplements

Psyllium husks (1–2 tablespoons at night before going to bed)

Standardized milk thistle extracts

Blue-green algae

If prone to constipation, try aloe vera

Antioxidants

Vitamin C (1 g, preferably as Ester-C, three times per day)

Vitamin E (286 mg per day)

Selenium (200 mcg daily)

Suggested balancing supplements

A vitamin and mineral supplement providing around 100 per cent of the recommended daily amount of as many micronutrients as possible

Evening primrose oil

An adaptogen, such as Siberian ginseng

Choose your own

Exercise of the day...

Complementary therapy of the day ....

Relaxation of the day ....

Indulgence of the day...

Mushroom, Garlic and Fennel Soup (Serves 4)

- 1 tablespoon extra virgin olive oil
- 1 large onion, peeled and chopped
- 3 garlic cloves, crushed
- 450 g (1 lb) chestnut mushrooms, chopped
- 600 ml (1 pint) semi-skimmed milk
- 150 ml (5 fl oz) Greek strained yoghurt
- 2.5-cm (1-in) piece root ginger, peeled and chopped
- 24 fennel seeds, crushed
- freshly ground black pepper
- chopped fresh parsley, for garnish

Heat the olive oil in a frying pan and sauté the onion and garlic until just starting to colour. Add the mushrooms and sweat for 5 minutes. Add the milk, yoghurt, ginger and fennel seeds and bring to the boil. Simmer for 20 minutes, then liquidize the soup until smooth. Season with plenty of black pepper. Garnish with chopped parsley and serve.

Spicy Chicken with Lemon (Serves 4)

- 2 tablespoons extra virgin olive oil
- 1 garlic clove, crushed
- 2.5-cm (1-in) piece root ginger, peeled and chopped
- 1 red chilli pepper, finely chopped
- ¼ teaspoon freshly ground cumin seed
- ½ teaspoon freshly ground coriander seeds
- 4 chicken breasts, skinned and boned
- 1 onion, finely chopped
- 3 tablespoons chopped fresh parsley
- 3 tablespoons chopped fresh coriander
- pinch of saffron or turmeric
- 300 ml (½ pint) chicken stock or water
- 1 lemon, sliced
- freshly ground black pepper

Mix together the olive oil, garlic, ginger, chilli, cumin and coriander seeds. Rub well into the chicken breasts, then place in an earthenware dish, cover and marinate overnight in the fridge. When ready to cook, place the chicken pieces, onion, parsley, coriander leaves and saffron (or turmeric) in a saucepan. Pour on the stock or water and bring to the boil. Simmer gently for 20 minutes. Add the lemon slices and cook gently for a further 10 minutes.

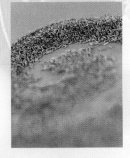

Remove the chicken pieces and lemon slices with a slotted spoon, place in a serving dish and keep warm. Reduce the sauce and season to taste with black pepper. Pour the sauce over the chicken and serve.

Balancing: day 9

On waking: Warm water flavoured with freshly squeezed lemon juice.

Breakfast: Fruit juice of your choice; mixed nuts, seeds and dried fruit muesli topped with semi-skimmed milk and live bio yoghurt.

Mid-morning: Banana and other easily digested fruits, such as oranges, apples, pears and melons, as often as you wish.

Lunch: Cooked brown rice; salmon tartare (this page); raita (this page); large mixed salad sprinkled with nuts and seeds; live bio yoghurt; carrot and/or apple juice.

Mid-afternoon: Mixed fruit and vegetable crudités, as often as you wish.

Dinner: Pasta with tomato and basil sauce (see page 124); large mixed leaf salad with lemon and walnut oil dressing; live bio yoghurt.

Evening: Fresh fruit as often as you wish.

Drink at least 3 litres (5 pints) of mineral water, fruit juice or herbal teas per day.

Suggested cleansing supplements

Psyllium husks (1–2 tablespoons at night before going to bed)

Standardized milk thistle extracts

Blue-green algae

If prone to constipation, try aloe vera

Antioxidants

Vitamin C (1 g, preferably as Ester-C, three times per day)

Vitamin E (286 mg per day)

Selenium (200 mcg daily)

Suggested balancing supplements

A vitamin and mineral supplement providing around 100 per cent of the recommended daily amount of as many micronutrients as possible

Evening primrose oil

An adaptogen, such as Siberian ginseng

Choose your own

Exercise of the day...

Complementary therapy of the day ....

Relaxation of the day ....

Indulgence of the day...

Salmon Tartare (Serves 4)

This dish must be made with extremely fresh fish.

- 225 g (8 oz) fresh salmon, minced
- 2 teaspoons freshly squeezed lime juice
- 2 spring onions, finely chopped
- freshly ground black pepper
- 120 g (4 ½ oz) live bio yoghurt
- 1 tablespoon wholegrain mustard
- 1 tablespoon honey
- 1 tablespoon finely chopped chives
- 2 tablespoons finely chopped dill weed
- sprigs of dill, to garnish

Mix together the salmon, lime juice and onion. Season well with black pepper and shape into four flattened rounds. Mix together the yoghurt, mustard, honey, chives and dill to make the sauce. Carefully place the salmon round in the centre of a plate, spoon the sauce over and garnish with sprigs of dill.

Raita (Serves 4)

- 1 medium cucumber, peeled and grated
- 3 garlic cloves, crushed
- 2 tablespoons chopped fresh mint
- 1 tablespoon chopped fresh chives
- 1 tablespoon freshly squeezed lemon juice
- 450 g (1 lb) strained live bio yoghurt
- 1 teaspoon honey
- freshly ground black pepper

Mix all ingredients together in an earthenware bowl. Season with black pepper to taste.

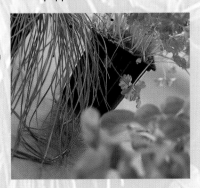

Pasta with Tomato and Basil Sauce (Serves 4)

- 2 tablespoons extra virgin olive oil
- 1 onion, chopped
- 2 garlic cloves, crushed
- 350 g (12 oz) beefsteak tomatoes, chopped
- 1 fresh or dried chilli, chopped
- 100 ml (3 ½ fl oz) tomato juice
- 1 tablespoon wholegrain mustard
- 12 black olives, stoned and chopped
- 6 tablespoons chopped fresh basil
- 450 g (1 lb) fresh spinach or wholemeal pasta
- freshly ground black pepper
- sprigs of basil, to garnish

Heat the oil in a frying pan and sauté the onion and garlic in it until beginning to colour. Add the tomatoes, chilli and tomato juice and simmer gently for 10 minutes, stirring occasionally. Add the mustard, olives and basil and simmer gently for 10 minutes. Season well with the black peper. Meanwhile, cook the pasta in plenty of boiling water until al dente. Drain and toss immediately in the sauce. Garnish with basil leaves and serve.

Balancing: day 10

On waking: Warm water flavoured with freshly squeezed lemon juice.

Breakfast: Fruit juice of your choice; kedgeree (this page); live bio yoghurt.

Mid-morning: Banana and other easily digested fruits, such as oranges, apples, pears and melons, as often as you wish.

Lunch: Jerusalem artichoke and hazelnut soup (see page 125); raita (see page 123); large mixed salad sprinkled with nuts and seeds; live bio yoghurt; carrot and/or apple juice.

Mid-afternoon: Mixed fruit and vegetable crudités, as often as you wish.

Dinner: Cooked brown rice; stuffed aubergines (see page 125); steamed spinach; live bio yoghurt.

Evening: Fresh fruit as often as you wish.

Drink at least 3 litres (5 pints) of mineral water, fruit juice or herbal teas per day.

Suggested cleansing supplements

Psyllium husks (1–2 tablespoons at night before going to bed)

Standardized milk thistle extracts

Blue-green algae

If prone to constipation, try aloe vera

Antioxidants

Vitamin C (1 g, preferably as Ester-C, three times per day)

Vitamin E (286 mg per day)

Selenium (200 mcg daily)

Suggested balancing supplements

A vitamin and mineral supplement providing around 100 per cent of the recommended daily amount of as many micronutrients as possible

Evening primrose oil

An adaptogen, such as Siberian ginseng

Choose your own

Exercise of the day..

Complementary therapy of the day ....

Relaxation of the day ....

Indulgence of the day..

Kedgeree (Serves 4)

- 400 g (14 oz) cooked brown rice
- 4 free-range hardboiled eggs, chopped
- 300 g (11 oz) uncoloured smoked haddock, flaked
- 4 tablespoons chopped fresh parsley
- 4 tablespoons chopped fresh coriander
- 4 spring onions, finely chopped
- 4 teaspoons garam masala or freshly ground curry powder
- 150 g (5 oz) live bio yoghurt
- freshly ground black pepper
- grated nutmeg
- freshly squeezed lemon juice
- watercress, to garnish

Mix all but the last three of the ingredients together. Pile on to a serving platter and sprinkle with nutmeg and lemon juice. Garnish with watercress and serve.

Jerusalem Artichoke and Hazelnut Soup (Serves 4)

- 450 g (1 lb) Jerusalem artichokes
- freshly squeezed juice of 1 lemon
- 1 tablespoon extra virgin olive oil
- 1 medium onion, coarsely chopped
- 600 ml (1 pint) vegetable stock
- 100 g (4 oz) roasted hazelnuts
- 2 tablespoons hazelnut oil
- 200 g (7 oz) fromage frais or yoghurt
- freshly ground black pepper
- extra roasted hazelnuts, crushed, for serving

Peel and dice the artichokes. Submerge the pieces in a bowl of cold water to which the lemon juice has been added to prevent discolouration. Heat the olive oil and fry the onion until softened. Drain the artichokes and add to the onions, together with the vegetable stock. Bring to the boil and simmer for 20 minutes. Meanwhile, crush the hazelnuts and blend with the hazelnut oil. Liquidize the soup, then stir in the fromage frais and season to taste with black pepper. Stir the hazelnut paste into the soup and gently reheat. Garnish with crushed, roasted hazelnuts before serving.

Stuffed Aubergines (Serves 4)

- 2 large aubergines
- 3 tablespoons extra virgin olive oil
- freshly ground black pepper
- 2 large onions
- 2 garlic cloves
- 2 beefsteak tomatoes, chopped
- ½ teaspoon acacia honey
- 1 tablespoon chopped fresh parsley
- 1 tablespoon chopped fresh coriander
- ½ teaspoon freshly ground cinnamon
- ½ teaspoon freshly ground coriander seed
- 1 tablespoon pine kernels or chopped walnuts

Preheat the oven to 180°C/350°F/Gas Mark 4. Cut the leafy ends off the aubergines, then place the vegetables in a large saucepan, cover with boiling water and boil for 10 minutes. Drain, then plunge into cold water until cool enough to handle. Cut the aubergines in half lengthways. Scoop out most of the flesh, leaving a 1-cm (½-in) thick shell. Lightly oil the inside of the shells and season with black pepper. Place on a greased baking tray and bake for 30 minutes. Meanwhile, chop the scooped-out flesh and set aside. Heat 1 tablespoon of olive oil and fry the onion and garlic for 5 minutes, or until beginning to colour. Add the chopped tomatoes, honey, herbs and spices and simmer for 15 minutes. Stir in the chopped aubergine flesh and pine kernels and continue cooking for another 10 minutes. Season to taste. Remove the aubergine shells from the oven. Fill them with the spiced tomato mixture and serve immediately.

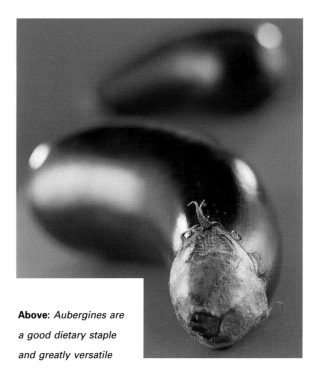

Above: *Aubergines are a good dietary staple and greatly versatile*

Future healthy eating

After following a cleansing and balancing detox diet, take care to reintroduce less easily digested foods, such as red meats, hard cheese and bread, slowly and carefully.

Continue with your balancing supplements for at least another 20 days, then stop the adaptogen and continue with the vitamin and mineral supplement, the antioxidants and the evening primrose oil.

Resources

Most of the following associations will supply lists of qualified practitioners. Telephone first for details and costs.

UNITED KINGDOM

ACUPUNCTURE
British Acupuncture Council
Park House, 206–208 Latimer Road
London W10 6RE
Tel: 020 8964 0222; Fax: 020 8964 0333
E-mail: info@acupuncture.org.uk

British Medical Acupuncture Society
Newton House, Newton Lane
Whitley, Warrington
Cheshire WA4 4JA
Tel: 01925 730727; Fax: 01925 730492
E-mail: Bmasadmin@aol.com
Website: http://www.medical-acupuncture.co.uk

AROMATHERAPY
Aromatherapy Organizations Council
PO Box 19834, London SE25 6WF
Tel/Fax: 020 8251 7912

International Society of Professional
Aromatherapists (ISPA)
ISPA House, 82 Ashby Road
Hinckley, Leics LE10 1SN
Tel: 01455 637987; Fax: 01455 890956
E-mail: lisabrown@ispa.demon.co.uk

AUTOGENIC TRAINING
British Autogenic Society
Royal London Homoeopathic Hospital
Great Ormond Street
London WC1M 3HR
Tel: 020 7713 6336
Website: www.autogenic-therapy.org.uk

BACH FLOWER THERAPY
The Dr Edward Bach Centre
Mount Vernon, Sotwell
Oxon OX10 0PZ
Tel: 01491 834678; Fax: 01491 825022
E-mail: bach@bachcentre.com
Website: www.bachcentre.com

CHIROPRACTIC
British Chiropractic Association
Blagrave House
17 Blagrave Street, Reading
Berkshire RG1 1QB
Tel: 0118 950 5950; Fax: 0118 958 8946
E-mail: britchiro@aol.com
Website: www.chiropractic-uk.co.uk

McTimoney Chiropractic Association
21 High Street, Eynsham
Oxon OX8 1HE
Tel: 01865 880974; Fax: 01865 880975
E-mail: admin@mctimoney-chiropractic.org
Website: www//mctimoney-chiropractic.org

CYMATICS
Dr Sir Peter Manners
Bretforton Hall
Bretforton, Vale of Evesham
Worcesterchire WR11 5JH
Tel: 01386 830537; Fax: 01386 830918

FLOTATION THERAPY
Flotation Association
PO Box 11024
London SW14 7ZF

London Flotation Centre
7A Clapham Common South
London SW4 7AA
Tel: 020 7720 4952

HERBALISM
British Herbal Medicine Association
Sun House, Church St
Stroud, Glos GL5 1JL
Tel: 01453 751389

General Council and Register of Consultant
Herbalists
18 Sussex Square, Brighton
East Sussex BN2 5AA
Tel: 01243 267126

National Institute of Medical Herbalists
56 Longbrooke Street
Exeter, Devon EX4 8HA
Tel: 01392 426022

HOMOEOPATHY
British Homoeopathic Association
27A Devonshire Street
London W1N 1RJ
Tel: 020 7935 2163
Website: www.nhsconfed.net/bha

Society of Homoeopaths
2 Artizan Road, Northampton NN1 4HU
Tel: 01604 621400; Fax: 01604 622622
E-mail: societyofhomoeopaths@btinternet.com
Website: www.homoeopathy.org.uk

IRIDOLOGY
Guild of Naturopathic Iridologists
94 Grosvenor Road
London SW1V 3LF
Tel: 020 7821 0255; Fax: 020 7821 0255
Website: www.gni-International.org

KINESIOLOGY
Association of Systematic Kinesiology
39 Browns Road, Surbiton
Surrey KT5 8ST
Tel: 020 8399 3215; Fax: 020 8390 1010
E-mail: info@kinesiology.co.uk
Website: www.kinesiology.co.uk

KIRLIAN PHOTOGRAPHY
Institute of Kirlian Photographers
51 Rushton Road, Kettering
Northants NN14 2RP

MASSAGE THERAPY
Massage Therapy Institute of Great Britain
PO Box 2726, London NW2 4NR
Tel: 020 8208 1607; Fax: 020 8208 1639

NUTRITIONAL THERAPY
Society for the Promotion of Nutritional Therapy
BCM Box SPNT, London WC1N 3XX
Tel: 01825 872921
E-mail: spnt@compuserve.com
Website: www.visitweb.com.spnt

OSTEOPATHY
Association of Medical Osteopaths
8–10 Boston Place, London NW1 6QH
Tel: 020 7262 5250

REFLEXOLOGY
British Reflexology Association
Monks Orchard, Whitbourne
Worcester WR6 5RB
Tel: 01886 821 207; Fax: 01886 822 017
E-mail: bra@britreflex.co.uk
Website: www.britreflex.co.uk

British School of Reflexology
Holistic Healing Centre
92 Sheering Road, Old Harlow
Essex CM17 0JW
Tel: 01279 429060; Fax: 01279 445234

SPIRITUAL HEALING
National Federation of Spiritual Healers
Old Manor Farm Studio
Church Street, Sunbury-on-Thames
Middlesex TW16 6RG
Tel: 0891 616080 (calls charged at 50p per minute)

TAI CHI
Tai Chi Union for Great Britain
94 Felsham Road
London SW15 1DQ
Tel: 020 8780 1063
E-mail: cromptonph@aol.com
Provides contacts, teachers, advice, books and tapes on the subjects of Tai Chi and Chi Kung (Qigong).

TRANSCENDENTAL MEDITATION
Transcendental Meditation
Freepost, London SW1P 4YY
Tel: 0990 143733

YOGA
British Wheel of Yoga
1 Hamilton Place
Boston Road, Sleaford
Lincolnshire NG34 7ES
Tel: 01529 306 851; Tel/Fax: 01529 303233

Yoga Biomedical Trust
The Yoga Therapy Centre
Royal London Homoeopathic Hospital
60 Great Ormond Street
London WC1N 3HR
Tel: 020 7419 7195; Fax: 020 7419 7196
E-mail: yogabio.med@virgin.net
Website: www.yogatherapy.org

GENERAL

NATURAL MUSIC
Sounds of the Earth
Oreade Music
E- mail: oreade@pi.nit;
http://www.pi.net/~oreade/home.html)

ORGANIC FOODS
Craig Farm
Dolau near Llandrindod Wells
Powys LD1 5TL, Wales
Tel: 01597 851655
Award-winning organic meat and fish by mail order.

The Fresh Food Company
326 Portobello Road
London W10 5RU
Tel: 020 8969 0351
Prize-winning mail-order suppliers of a wide range
of organic foods.

Organic Health
139-141 Ilkeston Road
Marlpool, Heaner
Derbyshire DE75 7LX
Tel: 01773 717718
Organic dry goods by mail order.

The Soil Association
86 Colston Street
Bristol BS1 5BB
Tel: 0117 929 0661
E-mail: soilassoc@gn.apc.org
Provides a directory of local box schemes and
home-delivery services for a small charge.

Organics Direct
7 Willow Street
London EC2A 4BH
Tel: 020 7729 2828
Award-winning suppliers of fruit, vegetables, dairy
produce and a wide range of fresh and dried food,
delivered nationwide.

Pure Organic Foods Ltd
Unit 5c, Eastlands Industrial Estate
Leiston, Suffolk IP16 4LL
Tel: 01728 830575
Suppliers of organic meats.

SUPPLEMENTS
Most of the supplements mentioned in this book
are available from pharmacies, healthfood shops
and supermarkets.

The Nutri Centre
The Hale Clinic
7 Park Crescent
London WIN 3HE
Tel: 020 7436 5122
Suppliers of the general, herbal and homoeopathic
supplements mentioned in this book. Mail order
service available.

Lichtwer Pharma UK Ltd/Medic Herb
Regency House, Mere Park
Dedmere Road, Marlow
Bucks SL7 1FJ
Tel: 01628 487780; Fax: 01628 487781
Suppliers of Ginkyo (standardized ginkgo), Kwai
(standardized powdered garlic tablets) and Kira
(standardized St John's wort).

Rio Trading
2 Centenary Estate
Brighton
East Sussex BN2 4AW
Tel: 01273 570987
Suppliers of catuaba, pfaffia, guarana and Super
Detox supplement (containing milk thistle plus
heather flowers and fenugreek).

UNITED STATES

ACUPUNCTURE
American Association of Acupuncture and Oriental
Medicine
4101 Lake Boone Trail Suite 201
Raleigh, North Carolina 27607

Tel: 919-787-5181

National Commission for the Certification of
Acupuncturists
Po Box 97075
Washington DC 20090-7075
Tel: 202-232-1404

Traditional Acupuncture Institute
American City Building, Suite 108
Columbia MD 21044
Tel: 410-997-3770

ALEXANDER TECHNIQUE
North American Society of Teachers of the
Alexander Technique
PO Box 517
Urbana, Illinois 61801 0517
Tel: 800 473 0620

AROMATHERAPY
American Aromatherapy Association
PO Box 3679
South Pasadena, CA 91031
Tel: 818-457-1742

AUTOGENIC TRAINING
Mind Body Health Sciences
393 Dixon Road
Boulder Colo 80302
Tel: 303-440-8460

BACH FLOWER REMEDIES
Dr Edward Bach Healing Society
644 Merrick Road
Lynbrook NY 11563
Tel: 516-593-2206

CHIROPRACTIC
American Chiropractic Association
1701 Clarendon Blvd
Arlington Virginia 22209
Tel: 703-276-8800

HERBALISM
American Herbalist Guild
PO Box 1683
Soquel, CA 95073

HOMEOPATHY
National Center for Homeopathy
801 North Fairfax Street, Suite 306
Alexandria, VA 22314
Tel: 703-548-7790

HYPNOTHERAPY
American Institute of Hypnotherapy
1805 E Garry Ave, Suite 100
Santa Ana, CA 92705
Tel 714-261-6400

KINESIOLOGY
International College of Applied Kinesiology
PO Box 905
Lawrence, Kansas 66044 0905
Tel: 913-542-1801

MASSAGE
American Massage Therapy Association
820 Davis Street Suite 100
Evanston, Illinois 60201
Tel: 312-761-2682

REFLEXOLOGY
International Institute of Reflexology

PO Box 12642
St Petersburg, Florida 33733
Tel: 813-343-4811

VISUALISATION
Academy for Guided Imagery
PO Box 2070
Mill Valley, CA 94942
Tel: 415-389-9324

YOGA
International Association of Yoga Therapists
109 Hillside Ave
Mill Valley, California 94941
Tel: 415-383-4587

FURTHER READING
The Shopper's Guide to Organic Food, Lynda
Brown (Fourth Estate, US & UK, 1999)

The 10 Best Ways to Boost Your Immune System,
Elinor Levy & Tom Monte (Bantam, UK, 1997;
Houghton Mifflin Co (Pap), US, 1997)

Miracle Cures, Jean Carper (Thorsons, UK, 1997;
Harperperennial Library, US, 1998)

The Antioxidant Miracle, Lester Packer & Carol
Colman (John Wiley & Sons, UK & US, 1999)

The Optimum Nutrition Bible, Patrick Holford
(Piatkus, UK, 1997; Crossing Press, US, 1999)

Starbound, Michele Wilburn (Starbound Enterprise,
UK mail order, tel. 0207 2481918)

Natural Energy, Mark Mayell (Three Rivers Press,
UK & US, 1995)

GENERAL
Allied & Alternative Medicine online database
(AMED)
http://www.rs/ch/wwv/rs/ds/amed.html

Alternative Medicine Homepage (University of
Pittsburgh)
http://www.pitt.edu/~cbw/altm.html

American Holistic Medical Association
4101 Lake Boone Trail, Suite 201
Raleigh, NC 27607
Tel: 919-787-5181

National Clearinghouse for Alcohol and Drug
Information
PO Box 2345
Rockville, MD 20847-2345
Tel: 301-468-2600 or 800-729-6686

Office of Alternative Medicine Information Center
National Institutes of Health
Suite 450, 6120 Executive Blvd.
Rockville, MD 20892-9904
Tel: 301-402-2466

Office on Smoking and Health
Mail Stop K-50
Atlanta, GA 30333
Smoking, tobacco and health information line: 800-
232-1311

Society for Nutrition Education
2001 Kilebrew Drive, Suite 340
Minneapolis MN 55425
Tel: 612-854-0035

Index

Bold type indicates a major mention of a subject

Acknowledgements

The publishers would like to thank the following sources for their kind permission to reproduce the pictures in this book:

A-Z Botanical Collection Ltd/83 Bubbles / Moose Azim 14/ Andrew Newton-Cox 12/Chris Rout 13 tl/ Loisjoy Thurston 54, 99; Carlton Books Ltd./ Susanna Price 75, 100/ Howard Shooter 5, 24, 25, 27,31, 39 tr, 40 r, 41, 44, 45, 47, 57, 59, 61 r, 115, 122, 123, 125 Cephas/ John Davies 89 br / Diana Mewes 90/ Mick Rock 26, 28/Stockfood

30, 62, 82, 120; Frank Lane Picture Agency/ David Hosking 110/ Chris Mattison 103/ 1an Rose111; GettyOne Stone/ Bruce Ayres 68/ Matthew Benson 113/ Christopher Bissell 94 bl /Andrea Booher 87/ Daniel Bosler 29/ Christoph Burki 40 l/ Michael Busselle 36, 121 br/ Peter Correz 18/ Chris Craymer 86/ Ron Dahlquist 91/ Deborah Davis 84/ Terry Donnelly 64/ Shaun Egan 34, 60 tl , 116/ Chris Everard 19 br, 37, 121 tl/ Stephen Frink 106/ Michelangelo Gratton 80 tl / Howard Grey 69/ Jaques Guilloreau 61 l/ Colin Hawkins 38/ Ian Logan 77/ Silvestre

Machado 118/ Alan Marsh 39 bl, 119/ Diana Miller 51/ Moggy 48/ Laurence Monneret 79/ Keith Morton 105/ Sanders Nicolson 80 br/ Frank Oberle 43 b /Dennis OÕClair 11/ Ian OÕLeary 19 tl, 70/ Andrœ Perlstein78/ Steven Rothfeld 92/ Kevin Schafer 66/ Ralf Schultheiss 112/ Rheinhard Siegel 50 bl / Richard H Smith 109 br / Paul Stover 58/ Hans; Strand 74/ Steve Taylor 43 tl, 50 br, 50 tr, 50 tl,69 br / Jerome Tisne 94 tr, 96 tl, 97/ David C Tomlinson 22/ Daryl Torckler 21/ Terry Vine 67; A Nelson & Co Ltd/108, 109 tl Science Photo Library/John Mead 8/Sheila

Terry 9 tl, 35; Superstock/6, 98; Telegraph Colour Library/Terry McCormick 32/ Antony Nagelmann 88/ S Rausser 93 tl; The Image Bank/ B Busco 72/ Gary Cralle 9 br/ Per Eriksson 81/ Macduff Everton 53/ Romilly Lockyer 22, 49/ David De Lossy 101/ P Ridenour 107/ Dag Sundberg 104

Every effort has been made to acknowledge correctly and contact the source and/ copyright holder of each picture, and Carlton Books Limited apologises for any unintentional errors or omissions which will be corrected in future editions of this book.